# Fast Food Globalization in the Provincial Philippines

# Fast Food Globalization in the Provincial Philippines

Ty Matejowsky

LEXINGTON BOOKS
*Lanham • Boulder • New York • London*

Published by Lexington Books
An imprint of The Rowman & Littlefield Publishing Group, Inc.
4501 Forbes Boulevard, Suite 200, Lanham, Maryland 20706
www.rowman.com

Unit A, Whitacre Mews, 26-34 Stannary Street, London SE11 4AB



British Library Cataloguing in Publication Information Available

**Library of Congress Cataloging-in-Publication Data**
Names: Matejowsky, Ty, author.
Title: Fast food globalization in the provincial Philippines / Ty Matejowsky.
Description: Lanham : Lexington Books, [2017] | Includes bibliographical references and index.
Identifiers: LCCN 2017046215 (print) | LCCN 2017047381 (ebook) | ISBN 9780739139905 (Electronic) | ISBN 9780739139882 (cloth : alk. paper)
Subjects: LCSH: Fast food restaurants—Social aspects—Philippines. | Philippines—Social conditions. | Globalization—Philippines. | Diet in disease—Philippines.
Classification: LCC TX910.P55 (ebook) | LCC TX910.P55 M38 2017 (print) | DDC 641.5/5509599—dc23
LC record available at https://lccn.loc.gov/2017046215

∞™ The paper used in this publication meets the minimum requirements of American National Standard for Information Sciences—Permanence of Paper for Printed Library Materials, ANSI/NISO Z39.48-1992.

Printed in the United States of America

*This book is dedicated to my wife and best friend Lorena Parker Matejowsky and our three wonderful children Bonny, Fletcher, and Griffin.*

# Contents

# Acknowledgments

The author would like to thank the following for their valued support and contributions to this work: Mario Granada, Josie Gonzalez, Hazel Gonzalez, Rubin and Letty Ang, Martha Heine, Emily Herrington, Jackie Rumberger, Charlie and Carolyn Matejowsky, Frank and Nina Parker, Lisa Haas, Jennifer Branson, and Dr. Tosha Dupras. Also, thanks to the University of Central Florida and Ateneo de Manila's Institute of Philippine Culture.

# Preface

I traveled to the Philippines in the summer of 2005 to examine the country's thriving fast food scene from an anthropological perspective. At this point in my career, I was just completing my third year as an Assistant Professor of Anthropology at the University of Central Florida (UCF) in Orlando. Newly pursuing the tenure track and anxious to reacquaint myself with the friends and contacts I had developed over previous stays in the islands, I returned to the Philippines with no small sense of enthusiasm. Indeed, this fieldwork session was not my first trip to the archipelago as I had visited the country twice before in the 1990s; actually living there for a year between June 1997 and May 1998. Since 2005, I have been back to the islands four more times in 2006, 2010, 2011, and 2015. Altogether, I have made seven trips to the Philippines for various research purposes and durations, ranging from a few weeks to some 12 months, since 1994.

I initially went to the Philippines in the summer of 1994 as a Master's student from Texas A&M University but not to study corporate fast food per se. With only two semesters of graduate coursework under my belt, I originally journeyed to the islands to ethnographically investigate the interplay between natural disasters and commercial retail trade. Pursuing this research topic proved worthwhile given the country's consumer market orientation and recurring impacts from extreme geophysical events such as volcanos, earthquakes, and typhoons. Looking back, my inaugural visit to the Philippines was life altering in the sense that it both confirmed my decision to pursue anthropology as a career as well as instilled within me a deep-felt appreciation for the country and its people that persists to this day.

Of all the reasons that I find the Philippines so endlessly fascinating, probably the most deeply resonant for me is the seemingly uncanny ability of Filipinos to co-opt outside influences, particularly those originating from the United States, to create something new and entirely their own. This propensity toward indigenization encompasses a wide variety of endeavors and undertakings. From the mid-twentieth century popularity of the live entertainment genre of *bodabil* that duplicates classic American vaudeville with a hodgepodge of sketch comedy, musical numbers, and dramatic stage pieces to the near fanatical devotion to a localized variety of U.S. basketball that is played professionally by 12 company-branded franchised teams within the Philippine Basketball Association (PBA) and throughout the archipelago on homemade sandlot courts by pick-up teams of shirtless young men in shorts and flip-flops (Bartholomew 2010), Filipinos demonstrate a real knack for reinterpreting and refining many tangible and intangible externalities into manifestations of local culture with increasingly tenuous Western roots.

Perhaps nowhere is this more in evidence at the community level than in the highly idiosyncratic and now ubiquitous mode of public transportation known as jeepneys. Every day these artistically imaginative public utility vehicles jam city streets in a colorful tableau of chrome-plated metal and customized paint jobs. With elaborate hood displays that feature a profusion of small mirrors, air horns, whip antennas, yoked miniature horses, and other quirky chrome ornaments, jeepneys offer a visual spectacle for passengers and bystanders alike. For commuters packed knee to knee along the parallel benches that face each other in back, jeepneys approach something akin to "mobile discos," especially at night, because of their booming sound systems and flashy interior lights (Garland 1998:24). In like manner, their dashboards and windshields reflect their owner-operators' distinct personalities, ornamented as they are with a mish-mash of translucent colored decals, tasseled fringe, and all variety of Roman Catholic motifs and imagery.

As flamboyant as these vehicles are today, their origins lay in a much more utilitarian purpose. Jeepneys trace their roots back to just after World War II when hundreds of abandoned or surplus U.S. military jeeps were repurposed in an effort to reestablish a transportation system effectively decimated by years of war. Over time, as this mode of transport caught on locally, the reliance on old American army jeeps gave way to imported or locally produced vehicles. Soon, a fleet of privately owned and aesthetically extravagant minibuses came to define urban transit in towns and cities across the islands, giving thousands of drivers and porters an economic livelihood as well as offering passengers an inexpensive way of getting around. Today, despite their initial U.S. military roots, jeepneys are now widely showcased as viable symbols of Filipino cultural identity both at home and abroad.

Doubtless, my status as an American with a notable fixation on all manner of U.S. popular culture has much to do with this abiding fascination on Filipino reimaginings of non-local influences. The oft romanticized funhouse reflections of American tastes and trends that I frequently encounter in the

Philippines, whether emanating from popular music, movies, television, fashion, or other expressions of this highly mediated realm, tend to emphasize the more superficial aspects of popular culture at the expense of many of the subtleties and nuances that U.S. audiences variously recognize and appreciate. Yet, this sort of indigenization is more than just pastiche. If anything, it is a highly discerning response to colonial, postcolonial, and neoliberal processes that produces new and novel forms that can be appreciated entirely on their own terms.

Indeed, as a nation of some 103 million inhabitants spread across three major island groupings (the Visayas, Mindanao, and Luzon), the country reflects an intriguing confluence of Western and Eastern influences. I should note that the Philippines is one of the few predominately Christian nations in Asia with well over 90 percent of today's Filipinos defining themselves under this religious affiliation. The vast majority of Filipino Christians, some 80 plus percent, identify as Roman Catholic, while the remaining ten percent or so belong to various Protestant denominations. Moreover, despite Tagalog (sometimes simply called Filipino) serving as the country's official language, the Philippines as a nation also boasts the third largest number of English speakers in the world behind the more heavily populated United States and India. The historical legacies of some four centuries of Spanish colonial rule (1521–1898), followed by a decades-long administrative and military relationship with the United States, are manifested in both profound and subtle ways at the local level.

As a frequent visitor to the islands, these influences are oftentimes entirely palpable. From the distinctive colonial architecture of the Spanish Imperial era to the considerable influence of the Roman Catholic Church, the lingering effects of this prolonged period of Hispanization remain an inextricable aspect of contemporary Philippine life. Similarly, the country's more recent colonial affiliation with the United States (1898–1946), however complicated or conflicted, continues to shape the lives of Filipinos. The introduction of an American-style public education system over a hundred years ago, coupled with democratic institutions of national governance based largely on those of the United States, exemplifies the Philippines' enduring linkages to America.

While these Spanish and U.S. influences continue to loom large, it is important to recognize that certain aspects of Philippine culture have also left their mark on contemporary American life, albeit in much less transformative ways. Perhaps nowhere is this more evident than in those seemingly quirky Tagalog terms that occasionally crop up in the American lexicon. Thanks in part to the everyday encounters of U.S. military service personnel with local Filipinos beginning in the late nineteenth century, a few memorable native words and colloquiums have found their way into the vocabulary of stateside English speakers. Indeed, I was pleasantly surprised to learn that words such as "amuck/amok" and "boondocks"—ones that I have pretty much taken for granted my entire life—are derived straight out of spoken Tagalog.

So, even as vestiges of Spanish and American colonial rule persist within the country's sociopolitical fabric, the Philippines still shares myriad characteristics with its geographical neighbors across insular and mainland Southeast Asia including China, Indonesia, and Malaysia. Among other things, these cultural commonalities include core social traits such as an instilled deference to family or the corporate group in nearly all decision-making activities as well as a distinct emphasis on maintaining social "face" in most, if not all, public contexts. At more tangible level for Filipinos and visitors to the country like me, local foodways draw notable similarities with the traditional cuisine and practices of its regional counterparts (see chapter 2). Filipinos' emphasis on rice consumption and similar modes of food preparation are but just some of the culinary practices held in common with neighboring populations.

While today's Philippines is certainly a reflection of its colonial past and regional geography, it is also something much more than the sum total of these enduring influences. To be sure, Philippine modernity defies simple categorization as the interpenetrative linkages between East and West produce a vibrant and textured cultural terrain that is as unique as it is complex. Adding further dimension to this cultural bricolage is the fact that some ten percent of Filipinos now live or work abroad as overseas contract workers (OCWs) or *balikbayans* (former Filipino citizens who are naturalized citizens of other countries and their children who periodically return to the islands). The financial remittances and cultural influences these transnational migrants contribute to their native homeland from places like Saudi Arabia, Dubai, Kuwait, Hong Kong, Japan, Taiwan, Singapore, Canada, and the United States lend an even more globalized character to contemporary Filipino identity, working to reshape the national tapestry in decidedly more intricate and unexpected ways.

Local foods and foodways are not immune to the transformative sway exerted by OCWs and *balikbayans*. In fact, their travels and time abroad make them powerful agents in disseminating preferences for new types of cuisine, food brands, and consumption practices to those friends and family back home with whom they maintain connections. The so-called "*balikbayan* boxes" that accompany these overseas Filipinos on their return to the islands have emerged as potent symbols in this regard, loaded as they are with all variety of non-perishable goods and consumables crammed within the prescribed dimensions of their cardboard frames.

Beyond such imported comestibles, the financial support of overseas Filipinos supplements household discretionary income at the community level to the point where many locals can now afford a range of consumer experiences that include regularly dining at American-style fast food restaurants. While never exactly tenuous, the financial and cultural clout wielded by OCWs/*balikbayans* over their communities of origin have only intensified as manifestations of social media and the Internet have become more and more ubiquitous locally since the late 1990s.

Suffice it to say, the Philippines offers anthropologists and others in the social sciences an ever-shifting topography from which to understand how global and local processes interface and influence each other. Accordingly, I returned to the archipelago in 1997 for a yearlong fieldwork session to support my PhD dissertation research. Somewhat more seasoned than I was as a newbie anthropologist three years prior, I yearned to immerse myself in Philippine culture in such a way that I could better understand the complexities, ironies, and ambivalences that characterize this arguably most "Americanized" of Southeast Asian countries.

Besides living in a local household whose members I now consider akin to family, I also endured my fair share of hardships recognizable to almost any cultural anthropologist who has ventured well beyond the familiar confines of home. Looking back, I consider these 12 months in the field as pivotal to my professional and personal development as I was able to collect enough ethnographic data to begin drafting my dissertation upon returning stateside in June 1998.

As previously mentioned, I did not focus on the local encroachment of American-style fast food restaurants in my MA thesis or PhD dissertation research to any great degree. Rather, in both studies I documented the commercial transformation of Dagupan City, Pangasinan, a tertiary city located on the main Philippine island of Luzon some 200 kilometers north of Metro-Manila along the Lingayen Gulf, as it rebounded economically from a devastating July 1990 earthquake. Dagupan's remarkable recovery from this calamitous event, in many ways, expedited the emergence of various modern retail enterprises throughout the city and across the northern Philippines. These highly capitalized ventures included several shopping malls, warehouse clubs, and corporate fast food eateries such as McDonald's, Kentucky Fried Chicken (KFC), Pizza Hut, and other brands familiar to Western diners.

For my PhD work I ended up contrasting Dagupan's post-disaster economic growth with the commercial experience of neighboring San Fernando City, La Union. I pursued this comparative research in an effort to better assess how natural catastrophes can accelerate pre-existing economic trends to the point whereby impacted communities undergo a dramatic surge of economic activity that would unlikely occur otherwise. Such analysis proved effective in highlighting the similarities and differences between these corresponding urban communities, rendering a more carefully hewn picture of post-disaster socioeconomic dynamics.

This is probably as good a time as any to raise an important point, one that will prove significant over subsequent chapters. Rather than concentrate my fast food research on one specific provincial Philippine community, in this book I follow a tack similar to the one I employed during my dissertation fieldwork. That is, I draw on findings from both Dagupan City and San Fernando City's local fast food scenes to document the sort of intricacies and incongruities underlying this dining format's spread and impact on local populations. This broad approach allowed me to take advantage of relationships that I had cultivated over the years within either city's retail trade community as well as add more ethnographic granularity to this fast food study.

Admittedly, during both of these early stints in the field (1994 and 1997–98), I ate at corporate fast food restaurants such as McDonald's and its homegrown Philippine rival, Jollibee, quite regularly. Whether in Dagupan, San Fernando, or elsewhere, this kind of patronage probably reflected the limited palate I had developed up to this point as a graduate student as much as it did the sense of comfort I derived from dining amid such ostensibly familiar and convenient surroundings. So, while I ate more than my fair share of native dishes, I also enjoyed frequenting quick-service eateries whenever and wherever the opportunity arose.

Truthfully, it was not that I intrinsically disliked or did not appreciate traditional Filipino cuisine. To this day some of my favorite local dishes include *pancit canton* (a tossed noodle dish with slices of pork, shrimp, and sausage), chicken *adobo* (a vinegar-marinated meat dish), grilled *bangus* (milkfish), and skewers of cubed pork barbecue. These native delicacies, coupled with a wide array of fresh fruits from across the islands such as *calamansi* (small lime-like citrus fruit), bananas, pineapple, and mangos, expanded my culinary horizons in myriad ways. No, what motivated me to seek out these corporate eateries was that, after consuming so much unfamiliar fare while living in a local household for extended periods of time, there were occasions when I simply wanted to eat something that I immediately recognized or that could in its own small way remind me of home.

Fast food restaurants not only provided a welcome refuge for me during those times when I simply wanted to decompress from the stresses and strains of my overseas fieldwork in somewhat familiar surroundings, they also offered a convenient setting for meeting and interviewing research informants over soft drinks or snacks in a relatively clean and cool environment. The ease and accessibility of these eateries allowed me to pursue my research agenda in various ways.

Plus, I found an entirely practical rationale for regularly consuming so much fast food. Despite a far–from-lavish food budget, my modest purchasing power as a fledgling anthropologist could still go quite some ways at these quick-service eateries, especially after the 1997 Asian financial crisis severely undercut regional currencies and effectively doubled the value of my U.S. dollars. Paying for meals and snacks at McDonald's and Jollibee quickly became my go-to method for assessing the general value of my American greenbacks against the Philippine peso. In many ways, I came to view it as my very own Big Mac Index, the popular metric introduced by *The Economist* magazine in the 1980s to illustrate how the standard cost of living varied by region vis-à-vis the pricing of this widely available and uniform global product (Ritzer 2004:7).

I suppose I was fortunate that my initial stays in the Philippines in the mid-to-late 1990s coincided with the first real wave of fast food expansion into the country's provincial hinterland. More by circumstance than design, I found myself well situated to ethnographically observe these developments as they unfolded in various ways at the local level. While restaurants of this type first appeared in limited numbers in and around Metro-Manila in the early 1980s, it took the better part of a decade before they gained a foothold in smaller regional markets like those of Dagupan and San Fernando City. Such growth was driven largely by the rising demands of a burgeoning middle class whose increased discretionary income and emerging appetite for the latest consumer products and experiences created new opportunities for fast food companies looking to attract fresh clientele.

As local dining choices in provincial towns and cities noticeably expanded, so too did manifestations of a previously muted global consumer culture. With the Golden Arches and its various national and international competitors carving out an increasingly visible presence locally, the street-level urban fabric of provincial municipalities began to take on a more cosmopolitan character. Regional urban centers, formerly characterized by neighborhoods of mostly drab low- and mid-rise commercial buildings, suddenly featured sleek new dining establishments whose signage, menus, and service formats contrasted markedly with most pre-existing restaurant operations. In just the three short years that separated my summer 1994 fieldwork stint in Dagupan from my yearlong research project in 1997–1998, the city's retail morphology came to include several new fast food outlets; some of which stood over two stories and offered consumer amenities such as children's playgrounds and banquet rooms replete with tract lighting and karaoke systems.

Given my penchant for hanging out at such quick-service eateries, I was able to encounter many of these new fast food offerings right alongside my Filipino counterparts. Looking back some 20 plus years later, it seems readily apparent just how instrumental this experience was in exposing me to new research possibilities. Although I could not really know it at the time, I was already starting to plot out secondary lines of inquiry that extended well beyond the original purview of my initial field efforts. After coming across a *Time* magazine review of James Watson's seminal anthropological edited volume *Golden Arches East: McDonald's in East Asia* (1997) while living in San Fernando City in early 1998, this potential shift in research direction seemed all the more promising. However unconsciously, I began mentally filing away stray observations about the local fast food scene or, in some cases, detailing consumer behavior or restaurant operational aspects that I found curious or otherwise noteworthy in my correspondence with family and friends back in the States.

As this material steadily accrued, it became easier to formulate the preliminary outlines of a new research topic that I hoped to one day anthropologically investigate. Doubtless, the germs of this book can be traced back to all those episodes of casual dining in Dagupan and San Fernando in the 1990s. My gradual tilt toward fast food proved all the more ironic in the sense that for years I had been repeatedly told, especially in my Texas hometown, that all that I could ever expect from an anthropology degree career-wise was a job flipping burgers at McDonald's. Yet, for a variety of reasons, the initial promise of ethnographically documenting fast food expansion in the provincial Philippines went largely unrealized for several years.

However poised I felt upon returning to the United States about building on the momentum I had established over my previous yearlong stint abroad, efforts to capitalize on this enthusiasm gradually stalled. As time passed, ideas of realigning my research trajectory toward a new topic of inquiry, much less returning to the Philippines seemed pretty much out of reach in the short term. Although family life and work obligations placed the projected next phase of my research agenda on the backburner, I still never developed second thoughts about the viability of this new ethnographical direction. Whatever type of doubts I may have entertained about branching out research-wise were soon dispelled following my participation in the annual meeting of the Society for Economic Anthropology (SEA) held in Decatur, Georgia, in April 2004.

With a thematic program organized by anthropologist and noted food scholar Richard Wilk, the meeting explored intersections of food, culture, and economy amid various global/local contexts. When the call for papers went out the previous fall, I figured that I had enough material from my San Fernando City fieldwork to cobble together a decent conference paper. I quickly drafted and submitted an abstract detailing how the city's burgeoning fast food scene emerged largely out of the complex interplay between both global and local capital. Several months later, I received word that my paper was accepted for the plenary session. With this welcome news, I finally began making genuine progress toward my goal of ethnographically documenting global fast food in the Philippines.

The SEA meeting turned out better than I anticipated. As a research forum, it offered a welcome opportunity for understanding local foodways through the optics of anthropological analysis. Three days of food-themed anthropological papers and a keynote address by Sidney Mintz made for a stimulating intellectual experience to say the least. Chatting with fellow attendees both before and after panel sessions proved no less inspiring. Like the official proceedings, these informal discussions invariably touched upon the centrality of food production and consumption in shaping aspects of various cultural, social, and economic processes worldwide.

If there was one thing the conference impressed upon me, it was the extensive appeal or intrinsic predisposition toward certain kinds of food scholarship. As a pervasive social phenomenon, it is difficult to imagine topics with broader allure or more personal meaning than food and foodways. There seemed to be a particular interest in papers like those presented during my panel session examining corporate fast food in all of its global manifestations. The sometimes curious forms that this dining format can take when launched overseas appeared to resonate deeply with conference attendees as most had experienced or been exposed to them while travelling or working abroad. While I am surely biased, it seemed that our panel session "Fast Food: Asian Appropriations" was among one of the best received sessions of the meetings. Alongside those papers detailing corporate fast food operations in urban China and Japan, my presentation on San Fernando City's recent embrace of quick-service eateries arguably struck a nerve with attendees. So much so, in fact, that our allotted Q&A time could not accommodate all of the comments and questions posed by audience.

Some of the more penetrating queries that came my way ended up exposing several blind spots in my research that I had not initially considered. For instance, I failed to address the political or postcolonial subtexts at play in the Philippines' prospering fast food landscape as the American restaurant giant McDonald's battles for supremacy against the more popular indigenous brand Jollibee just as I never sufficiently examined the role of wage earners in these new eating establishments. If anything, such gaps revealed a discernible lack of depth on my part. Certainly, they highlighted the need to broaden my research's future scope. Additional work clearly lay ahead; especially if I wanted to produce a more definitive account of fast food in the provincial Philippines. Taking these critiques to heart, I came away from the SEA conference with a newfound sense of purpose. More invigorated than discouraged by such constructive criticism, the meeting convinced me of the real possibilities of moving forward with a research agenda expanding upon this first foray into corporate fast food.

Some 15 months later, I found myself back in the Philippines pursuing this long-gestating research project thanks in part to some in-house funding from UCF. This 2005 summer field stint, followed by another one year later, not only marked a return to the islands that seemed long overdue, it also signified the beginnings of a new and more highly personalized fieldwork approach for me. I was optimistic about my research prospects this field session as food and foodways provides a viable context for anthropologists to participate in events almost as easily as they can observe them.

I felt there would be sufficient occasion to situate myself within the local fast food scene as both a consumer and observer. This favorable outlook proved prescient as I came to experience corporate fast food in San Fernando and Dagupan in various capacities over the next two months and again in July 2006. From a restaurant patron to a takeout customer, from a Jollibee birthday party host to an in-store survey respondent, I tried to capitalize on as many opportunities as possible to directly participate in this local retail sector. Ultimately such access allowed me to gain new insights and perspectives into how these quick-service eateries operate and how local consumers utilize them in various ways.

# Introduction

What follows is a decidedly personal ethnographic account of how corporate fast food has impacted local life in both large and small ways in Dagupan, San Fernando City, and across the provincial Philippines. Research findings, collected through a variety of data elicitation techniques including participant-observation, ethnographic interviews, and consumer surveys, tease out some new and compelling developments within this rapidly expanding commercial food sector. Admittedly, I draw mostly on my own experiences and observations while consuming fast food in the Philippines to add a distinctly reflexive dimension to this work (Ellis and Bochner 2000). What I have written probably best reflects an autoethnographic approach that conveys the particulars of corporate fast food in the Philippines through reflexivity and self-observation (Maréchal 2010:43).

In terms of organization, this book is divided into five chapters that approach corporate fast food in the provincial Philippines and elsewhere from various viewpoints and perspectives. When considered as a whole, information presented in these individual sections can be viewed as the constituent parts of an integrative and comprehensive account of the Philippines' thriving fast food scene; one that privileges data-driven empirical holism as a way to effectively delineate into a credible field account the quintessential multifariousness inherent to this seemingly ubiquitous retail format.

In chapter 1, I review much of the relevant sociocultural literature amassed over recent decades that critically approaches this style of dining both theoretically and ethnographically. Such an overview is useful as it helps situate my own research findings from Dagupan and San Fernando in a broader context. In chapter 2, I narrow focus to assess the historical development of chain eateries in the Philippines amid the persistence of traditional food and foodways. Of particular importance is the ongoing rivalry between an iconic global fast food brand and its more popular Filipino counterpart. In chapter 3, I turn attention to the experiences of Dagupan and San Fernando's respective fast food scenes that started to emerge in the 1980s. Such a longitudinal approach is not only helpful in tracing the rise of quick-service establishments in two distinct communities but also useful in showcasing the individuals and firms at the forefront of such efforts. In chapter 4, I explore intersections of children, families, childhood, popular culture, and chain restaurant operations within today's Philippines. In chapter 5, I consider the impact of corporate fast food on patterns of health, diet, nutrition, and obesity at the local level. In the Conclusion, I synthesize my research findings and offer some concluding remarks about fast food globalization in the provincial Philippines.

Interspersed throughout these five chapters are several personal vignettes documenting my recent encounters with McDonald's, Jollibee, and various other national and international fast food brands currently operating in the Philippines. I include these more reflexive accounts as a way to infuse some ethnographic granularity to this work and better delineate the sights, smells, and tastes of what it is like to experience aspects of Dagupan's and San Fernando's local fast food scenes firsthand. Undeniably subjective, these inclusions nevertheless offer detailed commentary about the foods and operational features of these increasingly popular eateries that could become easily overlooked in more conventional analyses. No less significant, such descriptive meditations offer something of a narrative counterpoint to the anthropological findings presented in the formal chapters they variously bracket.

In keeping with accepted ethical guidelines in anthropology, I would be remiss if I did not mention that some of the occurrences featured in the vignettes are actually a composite of several different events that I experienced over the years in the Philippines. I have selectively compressed these experiences primarily as a way to expedite this study's narrative flow while still effectively conveying the particulars of American-style fast food at the local level. Similarly, with the exception of my longtime research assistant, all of the names presented throughout this work that pertain to fast food happenings in Dagupan and San Fernando City, respective fast food scenes are in point of fact pseudonyms. This practice, which mainly applies to information presented in chapters 3 and 4, helps preserve the anonymity of those individuals, households, and family firms showcased herein.

Before wrapping up this introduction, I feel compelled to offer some clarification about why I am writing this book. Such elucidation is surely warranted given that readers have busy lives and, presumably, there are other things they could be doing besides reading about fast food in the Philippines. Without overstating the significance of this research, my motivation for anthropologically detailing local fast food retailing in both Dagupan and San Fernando City is based on three primary rationales, each of which is arguably relevant to students and scholars interested in understanding intersections of globalization, indigenization, and local food and foodways. When viewed altogether, a viable case will hopefully emerge about the efficacy of assessing corporate fast food's contextually variable impact on today's Philippines through the critical lens of ethnography.

First, the ongoing spread of corporate fast food worldwide vividly reflects the dynamics and tensions characterizing various global/local interactions. It seems that in early decades of the twenty-first century the global reach of corporate fast food is now all but omnipresent. The near ubiquity of this style of dining in societies across the developed world, and increasingly in less developed countries, makes for a compelling anthropological subject-matter in the sense that it both transcends global modernity while simultaneously revealing assorted idiosyncrasies at the local level. The overseas operations and menus of perennial global brands like McDonald's have been indigenized to the point where they have less and less in common with their American equivalents. While the service style and basic operational format remains largely the same, the production and consumption capacities of these foreign operations have assumed much more distinctive qualities. Quite simply, a McDonald's operating in Bithlo, Florida is in many ways similar and recognizable but certainly not identical to one operating in Dagupan City, Pangasinan or San Fernando City, La Union.

For anthropologists, the cultural terrain separating those universal features of corporate fast food from its more indigenized aspects represents an area rife with research possibilities. That is, it provides a viable ethnographic context for disentangling the sometimes complex interplay between macro- and micro-level processes in a way that is not abstract but directly resonates with readers. Since most, if not all, of us have consumed fast food at one point or another, the examples I present from the Philippines over subsequent pages will hopefully ring familiar to readers just as they will offer some revealing insights into how global culture is locally altered or manifested.

Second, as much of the sociocultural studies addressing the inroads corporate fast food has made beyond Europe and North America over the past four decades have been situated within one particular region, there seems a real need to expand the geographical parameters of this scholarship to better reflect the successes and setbacks experienced by McDonald's and its national and international competitors in other parts of the world. The scholarly work, thus far, compiled by anthropologists, sociologists, food scholars, and others on the worldwide advance of corporate fast food appears to share a territorial predilection toward urban East Asia (I will explore this partiality in greater detail in chapter 1). This Far East concentration is in many ways unsurprising, serving more as a reflection of the region's post–World War II economic growth than any deliberate disregard of restaurant operations elsewhere. Indeed, widening the ethnographic scope beyond the towns and cities of Japan, China, Taiwan, and South Korea to examine how corporate fast food operates in other locales, especially those beyond the developed world, would prove invaluable in both a comparative sense as well as adding more ethnographic depth to this growing research field.

Third, the current food studies scholarship, rich and varied as it is, has yet to produce a comprehensive account examining patterns of overseas fast food production and consumption from an anthropological perspective. A growing number of incisive ethnographic works have been published over the years in key peer-reviewed journals (*Food and Foodways*; *Food, Culture and Society*) and edited volumes (*Golden Arches East*) documenting corporate fast food's continuing impact abroad. These studies, however well-written and intellectually stimulating, nevertheless, remain rather constrained in terms of scope and objectives. Students and scholars seeking an extensive overview of how corporate fast food is locally manifested in communities outside of North America and Europe are still pretty much compelled to compile a reading list out of disparate scholarly sources. Adding to this difficulty is the fact that *Golden Arches East* was published some two decades ago, making a more up-to-date account of industry overseas operations all the more warranted.

To wit, this is something I encountered firsthand in Fall 2011 while putting together my syllabus for a newly developed undergraduate class, "Anthropology of Fast Food." As with my other UCF courses, I usually like to assign one or more ethnographies—the more engaging, the better—as a way to expose students to important anthropological concepts through more highly personalized field accounts. Arguably, nothing instills in students a deeper appreciation for cultures and lifeways different than their own than an intimate and well-crafted ethnography. For readers, even the most alien or superficially strange customs can approach the readily familiar when refracted through the critical lens of personal ethnography. Sifting through the existing food studies literature for some kind of anthropological work that systematically analyzes processes of fast food globalization in a specific overseas locality, it quickly became apparent that locating such an account would prove quite challenging.

Although I still consider the inaugural section of "Anthropology of Fast Food" a success and look forward to teaching future iterations of the class, I nevertheless think my students would have benefited from a more comprehensive fast food ethnography; one that blends a self-reflexive account of this subject-matter wedded to a rigorous anthropological analytical framework. So, for reasons that are partially self-serving as they would help fill a gap within my own class, and partially a desire to contribute something new and worthwhile to current anthropological food scholarship, I feel a book like this is now particularly warranted. Presumably, I am not the only anthropologist or food scholar teaching an undergraduate course where an ethnographic understanding of corporate fast food's varied impact on local lifeways would prove illuminating.

# *Chapter 1*

# Fast Food as Global Metaphor

## *Sociocultural Perspectives on Fast Food Globalization 1970s–2010s*

### VIGNETTE ONE: A PERSONAL ACCOUNT FROM THE FIELD, JOLLIBEE, DAGUPAN CITY, PANGASINAN, TUESDAY, JULY 5, 2005, LATE MORNING

Moving across the pavement toward the fast food restaurant, I pass under the watchful gaze of a giant cartoon bee. His sturdy fiberglass frame, burnished to a high polish, shines radiantly in the tropical sun like a veritable piece of Pop Art. Resplendent in a form-fitting waiter's jacket and bowtie, he cuts a flamboyant figure against the begrimed cityscape of multistory buildings fronted by utility poles weighed down with drooping tangles of black transmission wires. This larger-than-life character is impossible to ignore as he greets passers-by from his roost above the busy sidewalk. His bright costume and upbeat demeanor suggest nothing so much as a colorful fusion of Ronald McDonald's iconic brand status and the *Teletubbies*' waggish bubblegum appeal.

A gloved hand extends upward in a welcoming gesture of cheerful hospitality, while above two insect antennae mushrooms a white chef's hat. A small pair of translucent wings sprouts out of his sizable thorax making the prospect of flight all but impossible. His stinger is inflated to comic proportions and telescopes outward with alternating orange and yellow stripes. An exaggerated smile, bracketed by a pair of dimpled cheeks, tilts slightly askew, highlighting the rosy blush of his cherubic face. Altogether, this fast food mascot conveys a wholesome image of family fun that is as whimsical as it is unthreatening.

For many pedestrians, the campy charm of his jovial appearance registers no discernable reaction. They breeze past the statue as if consumed by more pressing matters. For others, the bumblebee's friendly countenance is just too

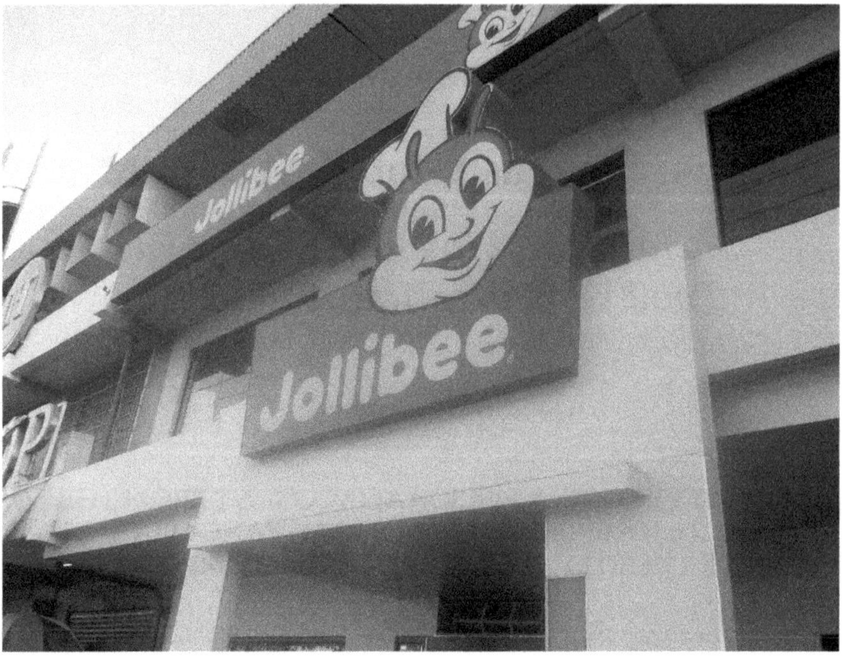


**Figure 1.1 Jollibee, Dagupan City 2015.** Photo taken by Ty Matejowsky.

powerful to resist. They stream toward the eatery alone or in groups seemingly at the behest of the oversize bug. Bypassing sidewalk vendors selling barbecued cubes of meat-on-a-stick, over-ripe fruit, and pirated DVDs along the way, their bodies brush lightly past me as they find their way inside. Intrigued, I cannot help but follow their lead to the restaurant even though I am not really that hungry.

A severe case of jet-lag has left my appetite in complete disarray. The natural rhythms of my eating cycle still adhere to their normal routine some half a world away. Until my dining schedule adjusts to its newfound circumstances on this side of the International Date Line, I will continue taking my meals whenever the opportunity arises. At the moment, however, it is not so much food that I crave but rather a short break from the relentless grind of Dagupan's dense urban environment. A disorienting barrage of street noises, strange smells, and sweltering heat works to unravel my already frayed sensibilities. With its modern façade and playful mascot, the eatery appears like something of a calm oasis amid the city center's dizzying rush.

The bee's saucer-shaped eyes sparkle with an impish glint as they track my approach up the steps to the glassed entrance. He presides over arriving customers with the spellbound aura of an enchanted Disney character. A few sprinkles of magical fairy dust are presumably all he needs to be brought to life. A security guard with a firearm strapped to his waist steps from behind the statue and opens the door for me saying, "Morning, *po*. Welcome to Jollibee." An automated door chime announces my arrival into the bright, climate-controlled eatery. A few tentative steps and I take a moment to enjoy the air-conditioning filtering out of a massive wall unit. Currents of cool air provide welcome relief to the oppressive heat wafting out of the city's concrete sidewalks and cinderblock buildings caked with layers of exhaust soot. Basking in the artificial breeze, I begin to soak up my surroundings with a keenly observant eye.

The Jollibee's modern interior is well-ordered and clean, as if sealed off from the chaotic street life outside. Pungent city smells of uncollected garbage and jeepney exhaust give way to the more pleasant aromas of grilled burgers and grease-laden French fries. Mealtime chatter and piped music help drown out the gear-grinding cacophony of the late morning traffic. The restaurant has all of the trappings of an American fast food outlet: trendy design, durable furnishings, and an easy-to-understand menu board. All of this I find comforting. I have only been in the Philippines for three days, after a seven-year absence, and the nagging effects of "culture shock" still persist. Slowly regaining my bearings from the jarring sensory assault that is downtown Dagupan, I feel like I have been transported to a place that is immediately familiar yet somehow alien.

The Jollibee bustles with activity even though it is not quite 11am. The dining area is near full capacity and no one sits alone. A glossy color scheme of primary tones highlights the smooth contours of the eatery's modish décor. Oversized photographs of fast food favorites as features of the natural landscape adorn the walls in neat symmetrical rows. The artwork's clever imagery depicts scenes like French fries as golden forests or ice cream sundaes in the shape of swirling mountain peaks. With sharp details and vibrant colors, the prints add a slightly surreal touch to the Jollibee's overall aesthetic. In this way, they perfectly complement the polished surfaces of the dining room's vinyl-laminate tabletops and chairs, radiating a warmth and style that is anything but understated. Curiously, the only adornments that seem out of place among the splashy furnishings are the small *Santo Niño* figurine that stands like an ornate doll on a small work table behind the service counter and the Philippine flag hanging discreetly over a side exit.

By all appearances, the Jollibee's floor plan mirrors that of a conventional fast food restaurant. From what I can see of the kitchen and counter areas, they appear state-of-the-art with numerous stainless steel appliances and accessories. The work space and equipment reflect a utilitarian design aimed at maximizing both employee efficiency and customer service. The nearby dining area is no less functional in terms of organization and layout. Gray and blue ceramic tiles patterned like a game board spread across the restaurant floor. Modular tables and chairs affixed with aluminum legs and no sharp edges are arranged in parallel rows, taking up this center eating section. A built-in counter running the length of an interior wall accommodates patrons atop swivel stools. I notice that these diners have to crane their necks awkwardly to see much beyond the colorful wall art. The fixed window tables on the restaurant's outer periphery offer much more in terms of a view. I can see a sizable late morning crowd take up nearly all of the dining area, leaving little room for lunchtime diners trickling in off the street.

Toward the rear of the eatery, somewhat removed from the main dining floor, stands the "Jolly Kiddie Land." A bi-level jungle gym, complete with a translucent tunnel system and safety netting, dominates this play area. The elaborate structure rests atop a spongy green mat and swarms with kids even though it is a school day. Most children comply with the house rule barring shoes on the play equipment. Footwear is stowed away in a plastic "sneaker keeper" located beneath a display of the playground safety rules. A few parents casually supervise their kids from the sidelines, leaving the more arduous daycare duties to a restaurant trainee. Close by, a cardboard cutout of the Jollibee mascot clutches a signboard with detailed information on how to rent the playroom for birthday parties and other events.

From where I stand, it is hard to get a fix on Jollibee's key demographic. Tables are packed with a cross section of Dagupeños including families with small children, text-messaging high school and college types, young professionals smartly dressed in *barong tagalogs*, and retirees flipping through tabloid newspapers. The sunburned Australian tourist in cargo shorts and tank top is an anomalous standout. I do a double-take when I spot two nuns munching away on fried chicken at a corner table.

Uniformed employees, mostly in their late teens and early twenties, dash about with notable alacrity. They clear tables, wipe down surfaces, and deliver food to customers holding aluminum menu numbers. When a group of nursing students begin rearranging seats to accommodate their party, Jollibee personnel move quickly to assist them. A neck-tied manager in short sleeves oversees their efforts. He holds a digital stopwatch in one hand and a plastic flyswatter in the other.

Lines to the service counter stretch back to the entryway. Customers file into the five or so parallel rows leading up to a register with only minimal space separating each. Queuing up, I study the numbered items on the lighted menu board. The majority of products are listed in English as opposed to Tagalog. English also seems to be the counter staff's language of preference when it comes to greeting customers. Even if the menu were entirely in Tagalog, I think ordering should be easy since it only entails pointing out my selection or uttering its corresponding number. A broad assortment of familiar and not so familiar meal and dessert options are available. The standard American fare of hamburgers and French fries are instantly recognizable. Less familiar are dishes with names like *Palabok Fiesta* or *Mais con Heilo*. Pictures of these more exotic items provide no real clue to their taste or ingredients.

Jollibee's wide product range is really quite impressive. It certainly dwarfs the limited bill of fare at the McDonald's I visited in Manila when I first arrived a few days ago. With so much to choose from, deciding what to get may prove something of a challenge. Hamburgers, fried chicken, hot dogs, spaghetti, and gravy-smothered burger steaks all have their own particular appeal. Luckily, the slow moving line gives me time to narrow down my choices. Playing it safe, I finally opt for the number three meal which is comprised of Jolly Spaghetti, a Yum! Burger, and a regular sized soft drink. A quick currency conversion in my head from Philippine pesos to American dollars reveals the price to be reasonable.

A heavy-set man in the line next to me, wearing a sleeveless Che Guevara t-shirt, basketball shorts, and flip-flops, starts up a casual conversation after I inadvertently brush against him. He seems to be genuinely surprised that I am in the Philippines, much less in Dagupan, and not visiting the beach resorts popular with tourists on the islands of Boracay or Palawan. The fact that I am by myself only serves to confound him more. Curiously, he is one of the few Jollibee customers unattached to a large dining party. In a manner that sounds more like a statement than a question, he asks, "You are American?"

"Yes."

"You are a missionary?"

"No, I actually work at a university back in the States."

He seems to ponder this a moment and then says, "I have many cousins who work in the States as nurse practitioners. They are in Virginia, New Jersey, and California. One is an X-ray technician."

"Yes, there are lots of Filipinos working in healthcare in the U.S. now."

"You know, it is the dream of most Filipinos to one day go to the States," he says, before asking "You are not there to celebrate July Fourth?"

"No, I was taking the bus up from Manila. I only arrived in Dagupan yesterday afternoon."

"Here in the Philippines, we celebrate Filipino-American Friendship Day," he says.

"Come again?"

"Filipino-American Friendship Day."

"Oh, that's right; instead of the Fourth of July," I say. "I think I've read about that before."

Our conversation is cut short when the customer behind him motions that he should move up to the register and order. When it is my turn, I am greeted by a young woman who is short of stature with a lively, expressive face. She wears a hairnet beneath her Jollibee cap and a nametag reading "Merly" is pinned to her uniform. Around her neck is draped a Jollibee I.D. lanyard bearing a laminated health card and passport photo. Her neat appearance and toothy smile radiates a vibrant glow of fast food professionalism. In a lilting singsong of Filipino-accented English she says, "Welcome to Jollibee, sir. May I take your order?" The earnest enthusiasm of her greeting takes me aback for a second. Unlike the poor or scripted service I often encounter at chain restaurants in the United States, she doesn't seem to be going through the motions. If anything, she seems genuinely glad to be waiting on me. I realize that this "friendliness" probably reflects her Jollibee training as much as it does her natural warmth. Yet, the authenticity of her "goodwill" doesn't really seem to matter at the moment. As a customer, I just appreciate the fact that her affability does not come across as transparently forced or artificial.

"Let's see. I'll have the number three meal."

"For dine-in?" she asks.

"Yes, for dine-in"

"And your drink?"

"Coke."

"Regular or do you want to upscale to large?"

"Sure. Let's upscale to large."

"Anything else?"

"No," I say.

Smiling, Merly places an orange plastic tray on the countertop and begins piecing together my order. Her cohorts at neighboring registers ring up orders with a regimented efficiency. Others draw fountain drinks or prepare frozen desserts. Work behind the counter moves at a brisk pace. Best I can tell, each employee is delegated a specific task in the food preparation process. All carry themselves with an urgency that suggests that they are understaffed even though by my count there are some two dozen workers moving about the restaurant. The pressurized atmosphere this creates inside the eatery is nearly palpable. It is as if the entire operation would grind to a halt if a particular task was not completed on time.

A Jollibee staffer busily prepares French fries to my left. It is a process fascinating to behold since he performs it with such seasoned proficiency. The teenager is clearly in his element as he submerges metal baskets of frozen potato strips into a deep fryer. After they emerge a crispy golden-brown, he dumps them into a stainless steel basin to drain off excess grease. With a deft touch, he lightly salts each batch before scooping them into preassembled cardboard containers. This last step is done with careful precision since every order is weighed for consistency on a small scale. Individual sticks are added or removed until the standardized weight is achieved. The fries are then propped between metal slates for easy retrieval. Each stage in this process is charted out on a detailed schematic that hangs above the fryer and closely resembles an airline safety card.

Further back, fry cooks with steel spatulas move beef patties around a sizzling grill-top. A Plexiglas barrier shields them and those doing prep work nearby from splattering grease. From where I stand at the head of the counter queue, the kitchen carries on with the mesmerizing aura of a beehive. Hamburgers are assembled as if on a production line with buns, meat, condiments, and other fixings put together in a series of controlled steps. Seemingly devoid of wasted motion, workers handle ingredients with disposable gloves to ensure proper employee hygiene. Once completed, burgers are wrapped in wax paper and sent down a metal chute for collection by the counter staff. The demand for burgers appears unrelenting. Staffers seem to take the fast-paced turnaround in stride. Many sing along to the store's sound system as they work diligently to fill orders. Crew members regularly glance up at the ceiling monitors displaying updated order information.

Merly has my order together in almost no time. The Styrofoam spaghetti box, wrapped burger, and plastic cup are laid out before me on an orange plastic tray. All bear the cheerful likeness of the cartoon bumblebee. It is fair to say that Jollibee clearly grasps the marketability of a high-profile, kid-friendly corporate mascot. Napkins and utensils are added rather sparingly to the ensemble when a shift manager arrives to inspect Merly's efforts. Peering over her shoulder, he nods to me politely while she works the register. If the supervisor's presence causes her any undue anxiety, it hardly shows. She seems to retain the same air of good-natured proficiency that initially greeted me notwithstanding her voice taking on a slightly more matter-of-fact tone.

"Sir, your total is 45 pesos."

I remove a yellowish ₱500 note that features the contemplative visage of national hero Senator Benigno "Ninoy" Aquino Jr. from my wallet and hand it to her.

"Sir, I have received 500 pesos."

Before making change, she holds the note up to the light to inspect its authenticity. Satisfied, she retrieves the proper amount and carefully hands it over with the receipt. "Sir, your change is 455 pesos." I am not entirely sure if her verbalizing each step in the transaction is for my benefit or her supervisor's. I suspect it may be a practice Jollibee uses to guard against allegations of short change from customers. I could be wrong but it seems that Jollibee harbors a subtle, if not covert, suspicion of consumers. How and why this is the case I am not really positive. As a customer, the scripted formality of paying for my meal, not to mention the presence of armed security guards and money inspection, feels vaguely out of place; certainly not in keeping with the restaurant's otherwise festive vibe.

"Sir, thank you for choosing Jollibee," she says, as I turn to find a seat.

Scanning the tables, I become acutely aware of the dining area's congestion. It is as if the real lunchtime traffic waited until I got my food to make its presence felt. My chances of scoring an empty seat straight away look pretty iffy. They appear even less certain as I amble up and down the aisles, clutching my tray, hoping that an available seat turns up. One or two circuits through the restaurant and I am all but convinced that no one intends on vacating their spot. When a table does finally open up some distance away, I am too slow-footed to claim it. A pair of schoolgirls, unencumbered by cafeteria trays, outmaneuver me to snag it. Even with only two of them and four available chairs, it is obvious that they really do not want to relinquish a seat. My overtures toward sharing the space are met with anxious grins and nods to their friends waiting in the counter queues. As I could have guessed, saving seats is not just a custom specific to the United States.

By this point, the futility of my search has gone from merely discouraging to downright comical. Worse, it now seems that the entire restaurant is aware of my plight. From my previous prolonged stays in the Philippines in 1994 and 1997, I know what it is like to be the unwanted center of attention strictly because of my foreignness. This is a feeling that I have come to terms with but never have truly relished. Sympathetic looks from the lunchroom crowd only heighten my sense of awkwardness. I realize that this fool's errand will eventually end in success. At the moment, however, I can't really see a way out of this increasingly absurd situation. Feeling every bit the outsider, I am quickly reduced to staking out individual tables. Diners now do their best to avoid eye contact as I mill about, anticipating their imminent departure. Several minutes of fruitless loitering elapse before I spy a couple exiting their window-side table. Seizing the opportunity, I move swiftly to claim it.

My efforts are momentarily delayed as a busboy clears away leftovers. Once he sanitizes the vinyl-laminate surface with a spray bottle, I table my tray and settle into the chair's hard contoured seat. The molded plastic is still warm from the previous occupants. Feeling a small rush of elation almost in spite of myself, I scoot toward the window to avoid the harsh sunlight streaming across the tabletop. Ensconced within a wedge of shade, I now have an up-close view of Dagupan's gritty urban terrain.

Downtown pulsates with a frenetic energy that is reflected both in the fake chrome of tricked-out passenger jeepneys aggressively vying for road space and the multicolored signage adorning the upper reaches of the city's modest skyline. Huge Jollibee promotional banners are slung across nearby roadways, and a garishly rendered depiction of Johnny Depp in *Charlie and the Chocolate Factory* is featured on one of the hand-painted movie billboard that stands atop the roof of an adjacent building. Looking almost like folk art, it is difficult to make out what other films these rooftop panels advertise since thick braids of electrical wires droop precariously over the parking lot and obscure my view. A row of orange Jollibee delivery bikes and several Toyota Tamara SUVs occupy the half-dozen or so spaces bordering the restaurant. Getting a car in and out of the lot without the assistance of a store security guard appears no small feat as the parking area runs up against one of Dagupan's busiest intersections. Downtown traffic moves in fits and starts through this chokepoint. Some pedestrians cover their faces with handkerchiefs to filter out exhaust fumes that tinge the air a hazy brown, while others clutch nylon umbrellas to shield themselves from the unrelenting tropical sun.

Inside, the restaurant's acoustics are such that patrons have to ratchet up their normal speaking voices in order to be heard. Overlapping conversations in Pangasinan, Tagalog, Ilocano, and English reverberate throughout the dining area, giving the space a slightly raucous edge. In the table ahead of me, a group of four young men in crisp *barong tagalogs* conducts what appears to be an impromptu sales seminar. The group leader punches figures into a pocket calculator while his companions look over a spreadsheet and sip coffee. Their discussion is briefly interrupted by a neck-tied Jollibee manager who discreetly swats at a housefly that has invaded their space. Unfazed by this disruption, the group continues on with their meeting once the pesky insect flies off.

All at once, a shirtless street kid of eight or nine appears outside my window. The boy looks down on me from his perch atop a giant potted plant that doubles as a makeshift ashtray-cum-rubbish bin. He knuckle-raps the glass vigorously in a bid for my attention. Above the collective din of the restaurant, I can hear him say "Joe" and "Cano" several times before he cups his hands around his face, pressing into the windowpane for a better view. These good-humored terms are frequently directed at American males and are doubtless remnants of the U.S. military's decades-long presence on the islands. The intense gaze of his rheumy eyes is impossible to ignore. When I tap the glass in response, he smiles and turns his palms upward as if asking for alms.

Instinctively, I want to help him; maybe slip him some food or money. At the moment, however, I am not really sure how to go about this. Do I abandon my seat and venture outside to give him some spare change or do I simply wave him inside for a quick handout? Before I can respond, the situation moves to resolve itself when a security guard approaches to shoo him away. The boy hops off the planter and scurries away, giving the watchman an obscene gesture once he is safely away from the restaurant. This episode would almost be humorous if it were not such a sad reminder of the harsh conditions faced by the Philippines' impoverished street children. With any luck, I can pass him some peso notes should our paths cross again.

Turning to my meal, I open the Styrofoam box and have my first look at the Jolly Spaghetti. Like fast food elsewhere, the actual product does not fully live up to its advertised image. The steaming pasta noodles are whiter than I anticipated and the sauce resembles nothing so much as watery catsup. Shredded white cheese and chopped hot dog bits add texture to the red sauce's otherwise diluted appearance. Taking a bite, my taste buds register a sweetness that is wholly unexpected. Instead of the zesty tomato zing that I normally associate with Italian food, the Jolly Spaghetti has a distinctly saccharine quality that is completely devoid of subtlety. In no small way, the sauce reminds me of the canned SpaghettiOs that I ate as a child. I make my way through about half of the order before the sweet taste becomes too much.

Next, I sample the Yum! Burger. It tastes almost nothing like American fast food aside from the white sandwich bread. The ground beef carries a sharp, peppery seasoning that lends the fried meat patty a serious Tabasco flair. With hints of garlic, onion, and, almost certainly, cayenne pepper, it packs a punch seldom encountered at U.S. burger joints. Surely, there can be no mistaking the Yum! Burger's distinctive paprika flavor with that of a Whopper or Big Mac. Sweet pickles, banana catsup, and mayonnaise add extra succulence to the burger's already juicy taste. Several quick bites and the Jolly Spaghetti's sweet aftertaste is all but cleansed from my palate.

Diners at neighboring tables really seem to relish the zesty tang of their hamburgers. Surprisingly, the seasoned beef lacks sufficient kick for some customers. More than a few generously douse their sandwiches with splashes of Jollibee hot sauce. Miniature plastic bottles of the red liquid are available at the restaurant's condiment station near the Jolly Kiddie Land. After procuring a bottle from the serving kiosk, I return to my seat and promptly uncap it. The aroma wafting out of the container smells potent. Tasting a few dabs from my fingertips, I am surprised to find the hot sauce so curiously underwhelming. By no means tepid, the liquid dressing is only moderately spicy, lacking the pungent intensity of American hot sauce brands. A more liberal dose on my burger, however, and the condiment assumes a more robust edge. The hot sauce really seems to come into its own as it complements the Yum! Burger's tangy meatball flavor with a full-on jolt of spiciness. All and all, there is little that I do not like about this decidedly Filipino take on the classic U.S. hamburger. In fact, I have to say that I find most of my Jollibee combo-meal to be high-quality fare; albeit curiously tasting by American standards.

As I finish up my Yum! Burger, I can't help but think of the scene from Quentin Tarantino's *Pulp Fiction* where mob hitmen Vincent Vega (John Travolta) and Jules Winnfield (Samuel L. Jackson) drive to a Los Angles apartment to retrieve a stolen briefcase with mysteriously glowing contents for their gangster boss. Ostensibly to take their minds off of the grisly work ahead, the duo fiddles with the radio, broods cinematically, and discusses the finer points of European fast food. Vincent coolly recounts the differences between European fast food and its American counterpart. Punctuating his tough-guy banter with the occasional profanity, he tells Jules that fast food in Europe is essentially the same as in the United States with a few notable differences: different names for the same products (Quarter Pounder with Cheese and Big Mac at U.S. McDonald's vs. *Royale with Cheese* and *Le Big Mac* at French McDonald's); different tastes and practices (French fries dipped in ketchup in the United States vs. French fries slathered with mayonnaise in Holland); and different menu options (soft drinks at U.S. McDonald's vs. beer at French McDonald's).

The scene is memorable not only for Vincent and Jules' *Men-in-Black* attire, crackling dialogue, and cocksure bravado, but also for its genius in conveying the skewed sense of place many Americans feel when dining at quick-service eateries abroad. Curiously, fast food seems to take on a deeper resonance when (re-)experienced in different cultural contexts. Certainly, the fast food model, developed and perfected in the United States over the past seven decades, loses much of its predictability for Americans as they encounter its global idiosyncrasies. Even subtle variations to this format can prove confounding to those of us for whom fast food has always been routine and taken for granted. Without question, the ingrained familiarity of American fast food provides only a rough template for negotiating the new tastes and protocols that these operations present at the global level.

In many ways, Vincent's fast food musings reflect my current state of mind. As an anthropologist interested in the effects of globalization on provincial Philippine communities, I find Jollibee, the most popular and successful Filipino fast food brand, to be particularly fascinating. The restaurant chain illustrates quite vividly how commercial forms originating in the developed West can assume new textures and shadings once they take root in foreign markets. Certainly, Jollibee appears as little more than the Filipino equivalent of McDonald's at first glance. A happy-go-lucky mascot, bright color scheme, and efficient service model are but just some of the features Jollibee shares with the global fast food giant. Where Jollibee really seems to distinguish itself from McDonald's operations in the United States, the Philippines, and elsewhere is in its distinctive menu and excessive courteousness.

It is easy to see that Jollibee provides customers a dining experience that is both fun and reflective of traditional Filipino values like family, hospitality, and playfulness. With a cooking style geared toward indigenous tastes and a product range nearly twice that of McDonald's, Jollibee cultivates a brand identity that successfully resonates quite readily with consumers. As a homegrown firm, Jollibee holds an advantage over its foreign competitors in determining what locals want in a quick-service eatery. At a time when many lament the spread of American fast food chains around the world, linking it to, among other things, emerging forms of neocolonialism, neoliberalism, and cultural homogeneity, it is intriguing to see Jollibee carve out such a vital position within the country's burgeoning fast food scene. If the firm's status as a national brand conveys any real drawback at the present time, I am currently hard pressed to identify one.

Having dined sufficiently, I feel almost ready to reimmerse myself in Dagupan's bustling street life. Since Jollibee lacks self-service beverage dispensers, I cannot top off my drink with extra ice or soda for the intense midday heat to come. In much the same way that napkins, utensils, and straws are doled out rather sparingly from behind the counter, free drink refills are a perk simply not extended to Jollibee patrons. It is probably no accident that Jollibee does not allow customer self-provisioning. Strict control over restaurant wares discourages notions that these items are somehow inexhaustible and free for the taking. Protecting supply stocks from consumer abuse is certainly understandable from a management perspective since it helps minimize both waste and operating costs. Yet, it also speaks to the subtle undercurrent of mistrust that seems to inform aspects of Jollibee's relationship with its clientele.

Getting up from the booth, I begin scouting out a disposal bin to dump my leftovers. The closest one is near the entrance, partially obstructed by a knot of patrons waiting for available seating. Advancing carefully through the crowd, I sense that I have committed some type of faux pas from the curious looks shot my way. This suspicion is promptly confirmed when a Jollibee trainee approaches to take my tray. He relieves me of the leftovers and says rather graciously, "Sir, I will be the one." Evidently, Jollibee customers are not expected to bus their own tables as they are in U.S. fast food eateries. The trainee empties my refuse into the receptacle and is off to other duties before I can thank him. As I turn to exit, the security guard already has the door propped open for me. An intense surge of heat and street noise confronts me as I step outside. Almost as if on cue, the young man says, "Thank you for eating at Jollibee. Come again."

Not knowing it then, I would return to this particular Jollibee multiple times over the next ten years in my capacity as both an anthropologist and fast food patron. Indeed, from 2005 onward, I witnessed various changes in the restaurant's operations, service style, and décor. This ongoing transformation proved revealing not just in the way it showed how Jollibee shrewdly responds to evolving consumer tastes in cuisine and amenities, but also in how the urban fabric of the surrounding built environment remains constantly in flux. Indeed, as neighboring retailers came and went during these years, the restaurant continued to serve as an enduring feature of the local cityscape, undergoing some cosmetic interior and exterior changes, but still occupying a central place within the real and metaphorical geography of downtown Dagupan.

## FAST FOOD'S GLOBAL UBIQUITY

Corporate fast food has emerged as one of the most conspicuous and widespread manifestations of global consumer culture. The company logos, distinctive color schemes, and kid-friendly mascots of popular quick-service eateries such as McDonald's, Burger King, Pizza Hut, and KFC are now instantly familiar to millions the world over. Like the uniforms and team insignia of Real Madrid, the New York Yankees, or other top professional sports franchises, these restaurant brands resonate with diverse populations across far-flung regions in ways that few other corporate symbols or operations can effectively approach. From Asia to Africa, from Europe to Australia, from North America to South America, the retail footprint of corporate fast food is as geographically vast as it is seemingly inescapable.

Within the span of some 70 years, McDonald's and its various competitors have left an indelible mark on contemporary global life and infrastructure; dramatically altering the built environments of towns and cities worldwide and transforming the street-level fabric of urban and suburban neighborhoods and vast stretches of highways and arterial road systems within these populated areas (Matejowsky 2002). Less concretely but no less importantly, they have also helped revolutionize established notions of consumer taste, quality of service, and lifestyle (Ritzer 1998; Ritzer 2001) to the point where customer expectations in various commercial industries and service sectors are now judged by standards of promptness and turnaround effectively pioneered by corporate fast food interests. The accelerated pace of global modernity, where sometimes "now" is not even fast enough, is in many ways deeply rooted in the world of corporate fast food.

So well-known are these quick-service restaurant brands internationally, in fact, that it is probably not an overstatement to suggest that corporate fast food now serves as one of globalization's most vivid metaphors. In both profound and subtle ways, this style of cuisine and the restaurants that promote it operate as something akin to symbolic shorthand for this unrelenting macro-level process that assumes manifestation across myriad sociopolitical, economic, educational, and media contexts. Indeed, the compressed (travel) timeframes, flattened geographies (real and imagined), and intricate webs of 24/7 (digital) connection that increasingly characterize the modern condition find distinct expression within the expansive milieu that is today's global fast food scene.

Like certain hit TV shows (*Baywatch*), blockbuster films (*Titanic*), pop music phenomena (*Gangnam Style* or *Despocito*), and other popular manifestations of the United States and global cultural industry, today's successful quick-service eateries help foster a shared consumer experience that deeply resonates cross-culturally. In this way, efforts at disentangling some of corporate fast food's intricacies and contradictions at the local level can elucidate important aspects of globalization's hegemonic influence over workaday life just as they can also reveal the ways global forces are variously resisted, refined, and indigenized by everyday populations.

Anthropologists, food scholars, and others within the social sciences have long been interested in understanding the construction, maintenance, and asymmetries of the global political economy through the prism of food and foodways (Mintz 1985; Phillips 2006; Wilk 2006). The historical and political linkages that define the prevailing world system arguably evoke a level of clarity and appreciation both within and beyond academic circles when critically refracted through the optics of food studies (Inglis and Gimlin 2013). Insights generated by such analysis have important implications considering how the production, distribution, and consumption of food informs so much of human social behavior and the development of institutions and hegemony across geography and time.

Indeed, the proliferation and popularity of American-style quick-service eateries outside of Europe and North America over the past 40 years is highly contingent upon the socioeconomic conditions fostered through policies of neoliberalism and free trade whereby flows of capital move between countries and markets with fewer and fewer impediments (Appadurai 1996). Corporate fast food's encroachment into the provincial Philippines and elsewhere in the developing world over recent decades owes much to processes of economic globalization which effectively extend the reach of industrial food and transnational corporations into previously untapped markets (Wilk 2006).

In many ways, anthropologists, food historians, and food scholars are ideally situated to critically examine the political and socioeconomic effects of globalization at various levels of impact. To wit, a rich and growing vein of contemporary food studies literature helps illuminate the macro-level processes of globalization and their local outcomes in both colonial and contemporary contexts. With few exceptions, corporate fast food bears notable similarities to other ingredients, (un)processed foods, and convenience cuisines that have variously transcended their historical and indigenous origins to achieve staple status within the variegated topography of the global foodscape. Just as of sugar (Mintz 1985), salt (Kurlansky 2003), chocolate (Coe and Coe 1996), bananas (Koeppel 2008), and ramen noodles (Errington, Gewertz, and Fujikura 2013) have, among other commodities, been embraced by millions the world over, so too has the signature fare of McDonald's and its competitors assumed an enduring presence within the dietary and lifestyle regimes of myriad populations internationally. The versatility, convenience, and allure exemplified by such ubiquitous comestibles not only traverse national boundaries, they also transcend social strata, giving them household status within the culinary traditions and practices of various echelons of society.

Today, intersections of corporate fast food and globalization within popular and academic contexts are so commonly encountered that they approach the undeniable. Since the 1990s when globalization first really started to capture the public imagination as the definitive hegemonic phenomenon of our time (Appadurai 1996), depictions of American-style quick-service eateries as compelling representations of globalization and mass consumerism have seemingly proliferated. Indeed, corporate fast food's glossy designs, distinctive menus, standardized production and service formats, and Western roots appear highly evocative within this global milieu, lending themselves quite naturally to illustrations of globalization and transnationalism.

For college students and other consumers of popular media, it seems photographs of non-Westerners garbed in "traditional" dress consuming burgers, fries, and soft drinks have become almost de rigueur features of anthropology textbooks, globalization websites, and various magazine spreads. For example, images like those of a Pizza Hut operating in out-of-the-way places or improbable foreign locales such as near the Great Pyramids or a Starbuck's within the China's Forbidden City derive much of their resonant punch from the juxtaposition of these ostensibly incongruous elements. Understandably, these pictures communicate succinctly much about globalization's sweeping influence and the corporatized contexts we now inhabit in ways that most descriptive texts can hardly approach. Such depictions retain a semiotic cachet and functionality that convey a good deal about the paradoxical nature of what happens as iterations of retail globalization take root in communities around the world.

## THE SYNONYMIZATION OF FAST FOOD AND GLOBALIZATION

To reiterate, few contemporary societies remain beyond the global reach of the fast food industry. Over the past four decades market conditions favorable to the expansion of corporate fast food have emerged throughout much of what was formerly termed the Third World. Thanks in part to the adoption of neoliberal policies that promote free trade and support economics of scale, McDonald's and its various competitors have been able to capitalize on the increasingly auspicious business climates of many previously untapped markets. The growing influence of a consumer-oriented middle class, coupled with a food service and production format that transfers easily across global settings, further expedites the worldwide success of corporate fast food.

These enterprises have become powerful agents in the spread of mass consumerism and Western values (Schlosser 2001:225–54; Stolicna 2000). Even for consumers who do not frequent these eating establishments regularly, it is now difficult to remain insulated from the industry's considerable sway. Commuters, shoppers, travelers, television viewers, and web users are all subject to the advertising campaigns, billboards, and restaurant signage of various national and international fast food chains whether they like it or not.

The proliferation of fast food outside of North America and Europe not only transforms traditional concepts of consumer experience, taste, and lifestyle, it also promotes eating habits and nutritional regimes that figure prominently in the rise of medical conditions like obesity, high blood pressure, heart disease, and Type 2 diabetes (Schlosser 2001:240–43; Sobal and McIntosh 2009).

Countries whose healthcare systems were previously oriented toward treating various maladies related to chronic under- or malnutrition now find themselves struggling to cope with the rapid emergence of these noncommunicable illnesses more commonly associated with Western lifestyles. In effect, these societies are fighting a two-front battle that cleaves largely along socioeconomic lines whereby those without much in the way of material affluence struggle with conditions stemming from not getting enough to eat while those from more economically secure backgrounds deal with the health consequences of eating too much (Popkin 2008).

Against this backdrop, it is easy to see how the synonymization of globalization and corporate fast food readily emerged. Such metaphorical associations are evident in various contexts, possibly gaining maximal expression within the more overtly political and activist strains of the amorphous global justice movement. Within these counterhegemonic spaces, where the asymmetries of advancing neoliberalism, international finance, and corporate power assume particular emphasis, fast food eateries typically function as nothing so much as de facto representations of globalization's more excessive and controversial tendencies. In this capacity, restaurant properties often become firmly positioned within the cross-hairs of those looking to contest, impede, or otherwise redress the far-reaching impact of globalization.

For instance, the street rallies against globalization, neoliberalism, and U.S. foreign policy that have rocked major world cities such as Seattle in 1999, Genoa, Italy in 2001, and Washington, D.C. in 2002, often entail the destruction of a McDonald's or some other fast food property. The symbolic value and near ubiquity of these eateries make them easy targets for protestors. Even the most casual Internet search of these protests reveals dozens, if not hundreds, of images featuring masked demonstrators venting their frustrations against the prevailing international political-economic order by spray-painting slogans on restaurant walls, smashing storefront windows, or engaging in additional acts of serious and petty vandalism. One wonders if it has gotten to the point where local fast food franchise owners must visibly shudder when their city is slated to host the next G20, World Trade

Organization (WTO), World Bank, or International Monetary Fund (IMF) summit.

Surely the most celebrated of these anti-globalization protests relate to the media-savvy exploits of French activist and current European Parliament member José Bové. His folk hero status in various progressive political circles is predicated largely upon the events of August 12, 1999, when Bové led a contingent of disgruntled French farmers in dismantling a partially built McDonald's restaurant in Millau, Aveyron. Their efforts, captured by a slew of news cameras, were staged in protest to new U.S. government restrictions on the importation of various locally produced agricultural products. Like some latter-day *Astérix*, the popular mustached comic-strip hero of Roman era Gaul, Bové's actions that day articulated the sensibilities of many left-leaning and nationalistic groups for taking a decisive stand against the encroaching influence of corporate fast food and, by proxy, globalization.

In many ways, Bové's actions echo those of Italian political activist and local food advocate Carlo Petrini, who organized protests against a McDonald's opening near Rome's iconic Spanish Steps in 1986. These demonstrations were instrumental in sparking the international Slow Food Movement which grew from mainly European efforts to showcase local culinary traditions vis-à-vis encroaching corporate fast food and industrial agriculture into a truly global campaign that has for nearly three decades championed grassroots initiatives aimed at preserving and promoting local foods and foodways. With some 1,500 local chapters or convivia worldwide, Slow Food represents something of an alternative vision or resistive counterpoint to the real and perceived threats of corporate fast food and industrial agriculture. In these ways, it serves as a viable rallying point for those promoting community and/or natural food production and consumption. To be sure, the Slow Food Movement owes much of its existence and enduring popularity to the varying levels of dissatisfaction that many consumers feel toward global fast food.

The synonymization of globalization and corporate fast food has an enduring resonance that pervades many aspects of Slow Food and the global justice movement. Such semiotic connotations hold similar currency within other contemporary domains as well, including, perhaps most notably, mainstream international political discourse. In this context, the unrivaled success of industry bellwether McDonald's is often used figuratively to inform those socioeconomic and political processes that diminish the effective importance of national borders and geographically bounded communities as well as seemingly compress global communication and transportation linkages to the point where the world feels decidedly smaller.

In the strictest sense possible, this propensity to couple globalization conceptually with the Golden Arches may simply entail the addition of an "Mc" to an already established term or concept somewhat like the well-known neologisms of "McJob," "McDoctor," or "McMansion" (Ritzer 2004:10–11). Whether used pejoratively or benignly, these so-called "McWords" closely resemble the "Cocacolonization" of years past which linked the now ubiquitous soft drink with U.S. foreign policy or America's hegemonic cultural industry. Such portmanteaus hold particular relevance as they suggest a uniform expansion of American-style consumer capitalism.

The concept of "McWorld" memorably used by political theorist Benjamin R. Barber serves as a prime example of this tendency. Barber employs McDonald's remarkable overseas expansion as a compelling substitute for globalization first in an *Atlantic Monthly* (1992) article and later in a more fully developed book titled *Jihad vs. McWorld: How Globalism and Tribalism Are Reshaping the World* (1995). The central premise of both of these works is that two macro-level forces—one rooted primarily in Western capitalism, the other in Islamic Fundamentalism—are vying for global hegemony in the early 21st century. The conflictive interplay of these opposing forces, he suggests, creates many of the underlying tensions that characterize global modernity during this particular historical era.

Unlike the mostly reactive and tribalistic "Jihad" paradigm, which promotes solidarity through a common religious-based identity, albeit one that frequently gives way to instances of intolerance and instability, Barber employs "McWorld" as a broad construct to describe how minimally regulated capitalism and the outsized political influence of corporate interests have developed over time to exert considerable sway over today's global landscape. Notably, he sees the efficient forms of production and consumption exemplified by McDonald's domestic and overseas operations as viable metaphors for this unabated global transformation. While Barber effectively gives "McWorld" the edge over "Jihad" in this lasting global struggle, he is critical of both worldviews as neither process does much to strengthen efforts at promoting real and lasting democratization worldwide.

Somewhat similar to Barber's "McWorld" concept is the one developed by *New York Times* columnist and longtime globalization advocate Thomas Friedman. In his 1999 book *The Lexus and the Olive Tree*, Friedman uses corporate fast food, in general, and McDonald's, more specifically, to illustrate how processes of globalization can help reduce the potential for military conflicts among sovereign nations. McDonald's figures prominently in this regard suggest that countries with the Golden Arches operating within their national borders are sufficiently integrated into the global economy. These countries tend to resolve their differences diplomatically rather than going to war with one another or as Friedman famously stated "no two countries that both had McDonald's had fought a war against each other since each got its McDonald's" (1999).

As a crude measure of geopolitical stability, Friedman's "Golden Arches Theory of Conflict Prevention" surely owes much to the so-called "capitalist peace theory" (Gartzke 2007) which basically maintains that it is not so much democratic institutions but rather expanding free markets that act as the prime bulwark against future military disputes among economically linked nations (Ritzer 2004:7). Friedman's theoretical fast food metric, which seemed to hold some novel validity when it was first introduced nearly 15 years ago, has since lost some of its explanatory power as several conflicts, including those pitting Israel against Lebanon in 2006 or Russia against Georgia in 2008, have effectively demonstrated. Despite such contradictory examples, the "Golden Arches Theory of Conflict Prevention" remains compelling if for nothing else than the fact that it reiterates the metaphorical potency of synonymizing McDonald's and other American-style fast food operations with globalization.

## SOCIOCULTURAL PERSPECTIVES ON FAST FOOD GLOBALIZATION

When considered altogether, the above examples do much toward highlighting the symbolic associations that have developed over recent years between corporate fast food and globalization. However much these linkages have assumed currency within the popular consciousness, in truth, they only go so far in conveying the sheer transformative effect that technological advances in communication and transportation, alongside the rapid socioeconomic integration of geographically distinct communities, have had on populations worldwide. While the global spread of McDonald's and its chain restaurant competitors certainly has resonant value in showcasing globalization's considerable reach, this kind of synonymization tends to fall short when it comes to delineating some of its more nuanced or subtle dimensions.

In many ways, the foregrounding of corporate fast food in this way serves to perpetuate a rather simplified narrative when it comes to understanding globalization's variegated impact vis-à-vis national and international quick-service eateries; one whereby the introduction of chain fast food restaurants into towns and cities across the developing world is essentially viewed as a distinct manifestation of "cultural imperialism" (Friedman 1999:21; Ritzer 2004:175–76; Watson 1997:3–5). Such thinking is largely predicated on notions that: (1) more affluent countries like the United States are unilaterally imposing their consumer tastes, market ideologies, and nutritional regimes on vulnerable local populations; (2) corporate fast food inevitably gives rise to increased global homogeneity whereby local foodways and other manifestations of traditional culture become subordinated to these external influences;

and that (3) developing communities are effectively incapable of counteracting or repelling the relentless forces of mass consumerism and globalization (Matejowsky 2006).

Even as such perspectives cannot be readily dismissed as baseless or far-fetched, this critical take on fast food globalization remains largely superficial as the launch of a quick-service restaurant in non-Western communities seldom occurs so simplistically. In this way, the synonymization of globalization and corporate fast food remains somewhat lacking, obfuscating as it does many of the more idiosyncratic dynamics characterizing the worldwide spread of this popular dining format. In truth and as will be addressed over subsequent chapters, rarely does the establishment of a chain restaurant such as the Golden Arches occur within a developing context without some degree of local receptivity or cooperation.

Far from being a one-sided process, the successful introduction of an American-style fast food eatery at the municipal level is largely shaped by the tastes, capital, and efforts of local interests. Most quick-service eateries would struggle to establish a viable foothold, much less actively thrive, within developing localities without adequately drawing upon such home-grown knowledge and resources. These local sources of capital often prove crucial in the spread of corporate fast food into the provincial regions of less developed countries. Their contributions to this transnational trend underscore the various ways in which the standardized fast food model can be adapted or altered to meet local demands. Along these lines, corporate fast food's global expansion probably has less in common with a strictly top-down approach whereby Western retail formats are unilaterally introduced into previously untapped markets.

A more accurate representation of this process likely entails some type of hybridization metaphor in which the interpenetrative forces of globalization and localization interface and influence each other in new and unexpected ways. The interplay between local entities and non-local corporate interests is of particular relevance. Even as Western populations may be inclined to take these restaurant operations for granted as their near ubiquity has become so closely intertwined with the fabric of everyday life so as to render them all but irrelevant, the same cannot really be said for those living in today's less developed countries.

While much of the brand recognition, technical know-how, and related aspects of fast food production and consumption retain their distinctly American roots when launched abroad, many U.S. diners would sometimes be hard pressed to recognize various other features of these overseas restaurant operations. From indigenized menu items such as McSpaghetti (Philippines) and the McHuevo (Uruguay) to distinct restaurant behavior involving the extreme rationing of customer supplies, coercive seating etiquette, and placing orders at service counters, a wide range of practices and perceptions concerning corporate fast food exists cross-culturally (Watson 1997). Accordingly, this increasingly omnipresent dining format presents a compelling framework for delineating how local norms and lifeways maintain their viability amid such highly corporatized contexts.

While it is difficult to deny that the Golden Arches and other popular corporate fast food brands now serve as potent, if not convenient, symbols for all that is problematic with processes of globalization and neoliberalism in select political and media milieus, these affiliations tend to hold less currency when considered within a more holistic purview. This becomes apparent when weighing through the steadily expanding body of social scientific work examining corporate fast food and its myriad socioeconomic implications at both the micro-level and macro-level. Using both theoretical and data-driven approaches, this scholarly research helps tease out some of the complexities and contradictions that characterize the operational idiosyncrasies and ongoing spread of corporate fast food across diverse cultural settings (Matejowsky 2007). If anything, ethnographic findings presented in this academic literature reveal just how much sway this style of dining now holds in shaping the everyday contours of global modernity (Ritzer 2001).

Social scientific analysis of corporate fast food extends back some four decades. Since the late 1970s, when cultural researchers first began to take notice and recognize fast food as a legitimate area of investigation (Kottak 1978; Jackson 1979), a growing literature on the production and consumption of this style of cuisine has been compiled. Anthropologists, sociologists, social theorists, and others within the overarching field of food studies (Fantasia 1995; Franger 1994; Kincheloe 2002; Kruèsteva-Blagoeva 2001; Ritzer 1998; Ritzer 2001; Beriss and Sutton 2007) have contributed to this emerging corpus of work. The fact that that many of these scholarly books and articles prefigure the mainstream success of well-known critical exposés such as journalist Eric Schlosser's *Fast Food Nation: The Dark Side of the All-American Meal* (2001) and filmmaker Morgan Spurlock's *Super Size Me* (2004) suggests that this type of sociocultural analysis addresses issues of real import and interest to scholars and general audiences alike.

When considered as a whole this scholarly research has produced some revealing insights into the degree to which our social lives and consumer expectations have been influenced or reshaped by the organizational principles of fast food (Ritzer 2004; Stephenson 1989). Sociologist George Ritzer's groundbreaking concept of McDonaldization (1993), in particular, has done much to illuminate the considerable amount of influence that the "rational" approaches championed by the Golden Arches and other quick-service eateries now exert over global modernity (Ritzer 2004). Although such changes have wrought all sorts of consumer conveniences in markets around the world, they have, according to Ritzer, likewise fostered an array of ill-effects including health and environmental hazards, attenuation of human relations, and the imposition of a new sort of "iron cage" mentality whereby the rationality of the imposed system begins to create numerous unintended and irrational outcomes (Ritzer 2004:28).

Similarly, this strain of fast food research has illuminated the increasingly transformative role that ventures of this type bring to bear at the state, community, and individual levels (Stolicna 2000; Watson 1997; Beriss and Sutton 2007). The fact that corporate chain restaurants have successfully made inroads in so many parts of the world (Norton 2000; Downie 2000) is doubtless one of the reasons that anthropologists and other social scientists find corporate fast food such an intriguing topic of scholarly examination.

Not discounting the merits of these scholarly works, however, it is erroneous to suggest that all aspects of the fast food phenomenon have received comparable consideration from social and cultural researchers. So far, certain facets of this trend appear to have captured more of the social scientific imagination relative to others. For example, nearly all of the anthropological literature on global fast food deals with matters of consumption; that is, how consumers conceive of chain restaurants, utilize their products, and adapt to the contexts they create (Bosco 1999; Watson 1997). Less ethnographic attention has been directed toward the role of production or the ways in which fast food outlets emerge, operate, and engage local markets. This tendency to favor the former over the latter makes sense as it is arguably easier for anthropologists and other food scholars to directly observe or experience aspects of corporate fast food by way of consumption rather than production. Yet, this research emphasis on consumptive practices, however compelling, creates only a partially complete portrait of fast food globalization.

No less significantly, there tends to be something of a geographical predilection for researchers investigating the globalization of fast food as noted in the Introduction. Although this is still a relatively recent phenomenon, most studies examining the social and cultural impact of quick-service eateries like McDonald's, Pizza Hut, and KFC outside of the United States and Europe focus on the developed nations of East Asia (Bosco 1999; Jing 2000; Noguchi 1994; Traphagan and Brown 2002; Zhongqiang 1999/2000). Anthropologists have especially trained their eyes on the introduction and success of fast food in the region's major metropolitan centers (Watson 1997).

That so much interest is paid to fast food consumption in the urban areas of Japan, China, South Korea, and Taiwan and not elsewhere is probably of little surprise. Unlike other parts of the non-Western world, the Far East has undergone a sustained period of economic growth over the last few decades that can be described as nothing short of miraculous (Terry 2002). This expansion has created conditions favoring economies of scale which have, in turn, facilitated the rise of national and multinational fast food corporations. This market climate has been largely absent in neighboring regions and elsewhere in the developing world until only more recent times. Hence, the previously limited presence or visibility of chain establishments in other non-Western societies has provided anthropologists and other food scholars with few real opportunities to study the effects of American-style fast food away from East Asia's major cities in any significant way.

Thus far, questions related to the spread of corporate chain restaurants outside of the developed world have not been fully explored by anthropologists. While the urban populations of East Asia are still recognized as important consumers of Western-style fast food, they no longer represent the only international market for this type of cuisine. Largely in response to an emerging middle class, state-of-the-art quick-service eateries are becoming an increasingly pervasive feature of cityscapes within the less developed countries of neighboring areas and beyond (Downie 2000; Lee and Karkoviata 2001; Norton 2000).

Millions of consumers in low-income countries now partake of this style of cuisine each day whether for breakfast, lunch, dinner, or snacks. As the popularity and influence of multinational fast food continues to expand across many less affluent regions, the geographical scope of fast food ethnographies has not yet broadened to address these new developments. Consequently, there are still aspects of global fast food that remain relatively understudied, offering anthropologists and other food scholars ample opportunity to examine them from various ethnographic perspectives.

A more holistic account of fast food's global impact, thus, necessitates expanding the boundaries of previous geographically framed research focused on Far East to those countries characterized by more marked socioeconomic disparities. Moreover, it requires balancing considerations of fast food consumption with those of production and examining the ways in which these dual processes complement or subvert each other at the community level. Such work would not only help elucidate the various ways in which global, transnational, and international trends affect and transform local communities, it would also contribute to current understanding of how such operations first arise within non-Western milieus. Similarly, it would offer a more nuanced interpretation of how local interests and tastes work to transform manifestations of corporate fast food into something more locally responsive and palpable. Finally, it would provide a rich opportunity for exploring the marketing strategies and operating procedures that fast food firms utilize to attract and serve populations with more entrenched socioeconomic inequalities.

Bearing such outcomes in mind, an anthropological account of the Philippines' highly profitable fast food scene holds promise for addressing some of the understudied areas of research mentioned above. Perhaps no nation is better situated to reveal the underlying challenges and complexities that characterize the ongoing advance of chain restaurants into low-income countries. Ethnographic findings calling attention to the considerable popularity of national and international quick-service eateries in the provincial Philippines would contribute much to this growing, albeit far-from-complete, body of literature.

By considering issues of fast food production/consumption alongside the local impact of McDonald's and its various competitors on urban life amid pervasive conditions of under-development, new insights into this globalizing phenomenon become more readily apparent. To this end, the next chapter traces the rise of corporate fast food within the Philippines over the past four decades with particular emphasis on the enduring rivalry between the Golden Arches and indigenous powerhouse Jollibee. Details about how these leading burger chains continue to vie for hegemony within this expanding market sector and the implications such competition has in shaping notions of post-colonial identity among various segments of Philippine society create a useful backdrop for understanding my ethnographic findings from Dagupan and San Fernando City over the past decade presented in later chapters. The distinctive personalities, operational successes and failures, and underlying political subtexts that variously inform today's fast food landscape in the Philippines offer compelling insights about national and international modernity that help reify concepts of globalization into something that is at once highly resonant and distinctly idiosyncratic.

## *Chapter 2*

# Of Burgers and Bees

## *Corporate Fast Food in the Philippines 1980s–2010s*

Since the early 1980s, American-style fast food restaurants have become increasingly intermeshed with the community fabric of towns and cities throughout the Philippines. The small number of quick-service eateries that opened in and around Metro-Manila's more affluent municipalities some 35 years ago mirrored their U.S. counterparts in key ways. These original outlets exhibited many of the hallmarks that Western diners have come to associate with corporate fast food including smiling uniformed employees, scripted counter service, standardized meal preparation, and sanitary dining conditions. Over time, dining establishments of this variety not only grew in numbers and geographical scope across the islands, they also came into their own in terms of cultivating a more locally responsive approach to fast food; rendering their operations all the more distinct from their Western equivalents in ways both significant and nuanced.

Perhaps only in the most outlying regions of the Philippine hinterland have such fast food manifestations failed to achieve pronounced visibility. In part, the country's insular composition of over 7,000 islands and a largely undercapitalized infrastructure have both complicated and constrained the ability of restaurant developers to establish a considerable presence in these more remote areas. Such limited prominence, however, is already beginning to change as the boundaries of corporate fast food's influence over Philippine society continue to expand with the ongoing encroachment of chain restaurants in nearly all corners of the archipelago thanks to improved infrastructure and mass media and Internet efforts that continually promote this global retail format.

While the Philippines' fast-food scene of today still bears a corresponding resemblance to what is encountered in the United States and elsewhere, it has now advanced to the point where many of its menu offerings and other aspects of food production and consumption appear decidedly homegrown. So much so, in fact, that these more indigenous elements can effectively obscure the more routine aspects of chain restaurant operations developed and practiced by McDonald's and other American-style fast food operators around the world. Clearly, indigenization efforts of this sort have played an integral role in shaping fast food's ongoing popularity in the Philippines.

It should be noted that the long-term success of corporate quick-service eateries was not a foregone conclusion in the 1970s when the country initially became subject to possible fast food developments. Despite the presence of various indicators suggesting the country maintained untapped potential as a viable overseas market for the Golden Arches and rival restaurant firms, the Philippines was still uncharted territory for those fast food companies looking to expand their global reach. A number of factors such as shifting demographics, an increasingly globalized population, and the entrepreneurial initiative of several key individuals and families all proved influential in helping these chain restaurant operations ultimately prosper nationwide.

The expansion of quick-service eateries out of bustling Metro-Manila neighborhoods and into the country's somewhat remote provincial regions over subsequent decades has not only altered the traditional character of local built environments, it has also steadily transformed prevailing notions about diet, consumption, and commerce among everyday Filipinos. The glossy aesthetics and cheerful corporate mascots showcased in the restaurant signage, logos, and other material trappings of McDonald's, Jollibee, and their various national and international competitors are now common features of cityscapes countrywide.

The convenience and consumer amenities offered by these types of operations are not only reflected in their clean and well-staffed restaurants but also in the jumpsuited restaurant employees who careen through workaday traffic on motor scooters to deliver food orders to hungry consumers. With so many trappings of corporate fast food now readily apparent in Philippine towns and cities, the overall effect of these enterprises is to effectively obscure any belief that at one time in the 1970s quick-service eateries were considered novelties.

In many ways, the rise of modern chain restaurants in the Philippines reflects the nation's increased orientation toward economic liberalization, its expanding middle class, and long-standing fascination with U.S. culture and consumerism (Matejowsky 2007). This avid appreciation of America permeates many facets of Philippine history and modernity including the contours of local foodways. After some 400 years as a Spanish territory in which the Roman Catholic Church exercised an outsized influence over so much of daily life, the Philippines came under U.S. colonial rule following events triggered by the Philippine Revolution (1896–1898), Spanish-American War

(1898), and American-Filipino Conflict (1898–1902). Besides establishing a public education system and representative democracy based in part on U.S. models, American influences also exerted a profound effect on (re-)shaping aspects of Filipino palates and foodways. Significant to this culinary transformation was the increased reliance on imported tinned food items manufactured and shipped from abroad (see next sub-section). As primarily dietary staples of American colonial administrators and Filipino elites, the consumption of canned products helped inform the Philippines' path to independence in the decades leading up to World War II (Elias 2014).

Beyond such historical developments, corporate fast food's ongoing popularity with Filipinos of various socioeconomic backgrounds also reflects how much Philippine society is subject to the transformative influences of an increasingly hegemonic global consumer culture. While the particulars of these seemingly unrelenting macro-level processes have been redefined in various ways over the years by local interests (Blim 2000), such indigenization efforts can only do so much in altering this fundamental shift toward a more consumption-based and brand-conscious economic system. For better or worse, the socioeconomic conditions created by this dominant market regime, where the privileging of capitalist accumulation and commodity fetishism all but predominates (Laurel 2010), have firmly taken root in communities throughout the non-Western world including those in the Philippines. These developments have, among other things, generated a market climate favorable to a wide range of commercial enterprises including new types of American-style eateries.

In order to more fully appreciate the particular sway corporate fast food holds over today's Philippines, it is useful to consider this popular fare within a broader historical/colonial and regional context vis-à-vis the emergence of local foodways and antecedent restaurant types. The next sub-section provides a cursory overview of some important developments that variously inform the character and contours of local dining both within and beyond the Filipino home. Focusing attention on this admixture of influences—whether emanating from the United States, Spain, Southeast Asia, or elsewhere—helps elucidate many of the conditions that ultimately paved the way for a now-flourishing corporate fast food sector in the postcolonial Philippines.

## THE PRIMACY OF RICE, COLONIAL INFLUENCES, AND RESTAURANT ANTECEDENTS

Like other aspects of local culture, traditional Philippine cuisine and food practices did not develop in a vacuum. These inextricable aspects of day-to-day life have been shaped in many ways by a diverse set of external influences that reflect the country's rich precolonial and colonial history. As mentioned in the introduction, everyday Philippine cuisine shares many commonalities with rice-based dishes prepared and consumed in China, Indonesia, Malaysia, and other parts of mainland and insular Southeast Asia (Van Esterik 2008).

In terms of both ingredients and eating styles, the importance of rice cultivation and consumption to regional diets cannot be overestimated (Ohnuki-Tierney 1997:166–9). So integral is this dietary staple to Filipino foodways, in fact, that its inclusion is often one of the primary factors in determining whether or not what is being served is considered a snack or a meal. This particular point significantly informs how Filipino consumers tend to view the status and substantiality of fast food cuisine. Many locals simply do not conceptualize the menu items of quick-service eateries as falling into the same categories as that fare traditionally served at breakfast, lunch, and dinner (Matejowsky 2008). As one of my Filipino friends told me, "Rice makes you feel strong."

Almost invariably, meals in Filipino homes feature servings of steamed rice alongside helpings of assorted meats and vegetables that are dished up from kitchen bowls covered by ventilated plastic lids to keep flies away. At dinnertime, families generally eat together around tables adorned with colorful vinyl tablecloths and rotating trays or Lazy Susans full of condiments and seasonings. Servings are typically scooped out of dishes and onto plates with wooden or plastic spoons. Meals are then consumed with either hands or utensils. Unlike in the United States where knives and forks hold prominence, spoons and forks tend to be the most commonly employed utensils at Filipino dinner tables. It is quite easy to maneuver rice and other foods onto a fork with the help of a spoon. Speaking personally, I never really got used to eating with my hands even though on those occasions when I did it seemed to greatly please my Filipino hosts and earn me some measure of credibility and goodwill.

Among everyday Filipino families, cooking, food provisioning, and grocery shopping is rarely the purview of anyone but working and stay-at-home mothers/wives or other female household members. Fresh fruits and vegetables are typically purchased each day by these females from various wet markets located in and around urban centers. Other items such as canned and powdered goods, soft drinks, packaged snacks, and the like are bought less frequently from various modern supermarkets or small neighborhood sari-sari ("variety") stores. In these latter establishments, merchandise can almost always be acquired on credit. Such normative gender roles whereby females perform most food-related tasks persist across various social strata even as more women work outside the home. That said, among affluent and moderately well-off families—particularly Chinese-Filipino households—meal preparation is often performed by hired female help. In many cases, these domestic workers are elderly Filipinas who live with families in small quarters and receive modest wages for their work.

In terms of how home-cooked meals are prepared among most everyday Filipinos, stovetop cooking, as opposed to baking or oven-use, tends to be the most widespread method. While less impoverished families may have store bought kitchen appliances like microwaves and/or electric and gas ranges at their disposal, poor and working poor households generally rely on either small charcoal ovens or utilitarian stovetops that most Westerners would associate with no-frills camping stoves. These latter devices are fueled by exchangeable propane tanks that are widely available in both rural and urban settings. Many evenings, I would encounter friends and neighbors riding as passengers on hired tri-bikes (bicycle taxis with welded-on sidecars) on the way back from the local propane dealer to replace a recently depleted gas tank with a full container.

Given this primary mode of meal preparation, many main dishes served in local households feature meats, fish, or poultry fried in cooking oil. Small plastic bags filled with this cooking essential are sold for one or two pesos at most sari-sari stores at the neighborhood level. Besides these gas stoves, nearly all Filipino kitchens feature rice cookers that most Americans would recognize as resembling crockpots. These timed pressure cookers provide a convenient and economical way of preparing this enduring staple item throughout the Philippines and Southeast Asia.

Beyond the long-standing primacy of rice in today's Philippines, there are also myriad types of fruit, pork, poultry, and fish preparations, not to mention a whole slew of prepared snacks or street foods, which effectively mirror what can be found in towns and cities across Southeast Asia. Like other countries in this part of the world, the Philippines maintains a vibrant street food scene that continues to thrive even with ongoing encroachment of corporate fast food at the local level. Whether operating along bustling city sidewalks or hawking items within temporary urban markets, ambulant and semi-stationary food sellers comprise a vital segment of local street economies. From the enduring popularity of partially incubated duck eggs (Matejowsky 2013) to long-standing preferences for mangoes and sticky rice dishes (Van Esterik 2008), culinary mainstays like these help perpetuate a basic regional style of street cuisine that can become somewhat less homogenous as geographical focus narrows to particular countries or provinces. Despite such discontinuities at the national and local levels, the food culture of Southeast Asia retains sufficient culinary coherence so as to be readily identifiable when comparing it to its regional counterparts from other parts of the globe.

While rice's centrality to native Filipino diets doubtless owes as much to the country's particular geography and tropical climate as it does to historical links to populations living in neighboring regions and beyond, other food preferences are more directly the result of Western colonialism. Some four centuries of Hispanic hegemony (1521–1898) over the islands left an indelible mark on nearly all areas of social and cultural life including local foodways. The Spanish influence on the way Filipinos conceptualize and consume food became so sufficiently indigenized at the community level so as to now be firmly entrenched in local households.

Besides the introduction of key vegetables such as mais (corn) and meat staples like longganisa (sausage) into native foodways, Spanish colonizers also helped institute the popular late-afternoon snack time known as *merienda* as an integral aspect of workaday life. Not unlike British teatime, *merienda* is basically a time to socialize with friends, coworkers, or classmates over beverages like coffee and usually some type of sweet or savory fare. As will be discussed later, the social opportunities afforded by *merienda* lend themselves quite well to the informality and convenience associated with American-style fast food restaurants.

In no small way, the integration of outside culinary influences to Filipino palates and dining practices intensified during the American colonial period which lasted for nearly half a century after the 1898 Spanish-American War. It was during the decades leading up to and just after World War II when the impact of industrialized foods became more readily appreciable at the local level (Elias 2014).

Canned and processed foods such as SPAM, sardines, and corn beef assumed a newfound prominence in the culinary lives of affluent and moderately affluent Filipinos before eventually becoming more prevalent across less well-off socioeconomic strata (Cordero-Fernando 1992). The appeal of such non-perishable items is certainly understandable seeing as most homes at the time lacked proper refrigeration or electricity. This long shelf life, coupled with the products' easy preparation, made them ideal for households both rich and poor throughout the archipelago. So much so, in fact, that these tinned foods continue to exhibit an impressive staying power decades after their initial introduction (Matejowsky 2007). The centrality of such fare within everyday Filipino foodways almost rivals that of steamed rice. As my longtime research assistant Mario told me, "All Filipinos need to exist is coffee, rice, and canned sardines."

It was also during the American period or soon thereafter when dining out at sit-down restaurants became an increasingly common pastime. This was particularly the case for those urbanites with some material prosperity living in and around Manila and other large cities (Cordero-Fernando 1976). Unlike the still prevalent street canteens or carinderias, where students, commuters, office workers, and others can choose from assorted cauldrons of affordable viands served turo-turo ("point-point") style for either take-out or on-site consumption, these new types of dining venues offered locals a range of consumer amenities and menu options heretofore largely unavailable. Whether such restaurants were mom-and-pop coffee shops, ice cream parlors, Chinese restaurants, or American-style diners, they usually presented some modest degree of sophistication (e.g., wait or counter staff, tablecloths, and cutlery) or improved sanitation (e.g., on-premises wash stations and restrooms) that was largely absent in these earlier and more no-frills eateries.

In many respects, it is easy to see how the increased number of sit-down restaurants blossomed alongside the expansion of the country's postwar retail economy where growing numbers of urban Filipinos had newfound disposable income (Cordero-Fernando 1976). A few eateries became so popular with urban diners in and around Metro-Manila during this time that branches soon began to appear in other Philippine towns and cities. Two prominent examples of this trend are Max's of Manila, popularly known as Max's Restaurant or Max's Chicken, and Goldilocks Bakeshop. The former is a sit-down restaurant known for its wide selection of fried chicken and traditional Filipino cuisine, while the latter is a bakery that offers cakes and other confections alongside lunch and dinner items served turo-turo style. Incidentally, one of the first restaurant meals I ever consumed in the Philippines was at Max's Chicken in May 1994 during a stopover in Tarlac City, Tarlac on the six-hour bus ride from Metro-Manila to Dagupan City. Beyond really liking the fried chicken, I remember finding the pinkabet (indigenous vegetable dish) too bitter to eat.

Both Max's and Goldilocks have cultivated distinct consumer followings with a mainly middle- and upper-class clientele over the years even as they remain popular household names among Filipinos of all socioeconomic strata. Max's commenced operations in 1945 and currently operates some 150 eateries across the islands and even a few in North America including ones in California and New Jersey. Goldilocks started as a mom-and-pop bakery in 1966 that proved so popular with consumers that it soon began expanding its operational reach both domestically and internationally. In the United States, Goldilocks locations can be found in Las Vegas, San Francisco, and San Jose. Indeed, rare is the secondary or tertiary city in today's Philippines that does not possess one or more Max's or Goldilocks restaurants. Several shopping malls in both Dagupan and San Fernando City feature Goldilocks outlets while only San Fernando has a Max's Restaurant on the highway leading into town.

Perhaps more abstractly but arguably no less influential in the development of Filipino foodways during the U.S. colonial period and beyond is an enduring attraction with nearly all things American. For many Filipinos, the products, personalities, and lifestyles promoted by American manufacturers and the U.S. cultural industry continue to exert a powerful allure that even sporadic geopolitical differences between the two countries cannot readily dislodge. Indeed, locals seem to harbor intense feelings of admiration or at the very least a discernable appreciation for the material and cultural goods originating from across the Pacific. Such positive associations continue to loom large over the Filipino imagination even as they tend to reflect more superficial or romanticized aspects of a largely imagined "U.S.A." than anything that is actually grounded in the day-to-day realities of American modernity (Matejowsky 2007).

This abiding fascination with American culture arguably finds expression in the ongoing development of the Philippines' national fast-food scene. In both profound and subtle ways, Filipinos' orientation toward the United States made the introduction of new American-style fast-food operations and cuisine into local lifeways all the more viable. Unlike other foreign markets where indigenous consumers were less familiar with the particulars of quick-service eateries and their attendant dining forms and customs, the Philippines was more ideally situated when it came to understanding and accepting manifestations of corporate fast food given the country's long-standing relationship with the United States.

The fact that the country was home to two of the largest American overseas military installations—U.S. Naval Base Subic Bay and Clark Air Base—throughout the Cold War period made such sentiments arguably even more appreciable. If anything, it is surprising that McDonald's and other global fast food brands did not establish a market presence within the country sooner given the postcolonial ties between the Philippines and the United States. While the Golden Arches launched its first Far East restaurant operation in Japan in 1971, it would be some ten years before the company finally entered the Philippines.

## MCDONALD'S AND JOLLIBEE

With some 35 years hindsight, it is probably no exaggeration to suggest that corporate fast food has sufficiently captured the imaginations and tastes of Filipinos throughout the archipelago. Fast food appetites have grown almost exponentially following McDonald's official launch in 1981. Since this time numerous transnational chains including A&W, Burger King, Dunkin' Donuts, Domino's, KFC, Pizza Hut, Kenny Rogers' Roasters, and Wendy's have opened outlets across the islands. These eateries alongside their home-grown counterparts of Chowking, Greenwich Pizza, Goldilocks Bakeshop, and Shakey's Pizza gave many Filipinos their first taste of an American-style fast food dining experience.

By the beginning of the 21st century, dining out at chain restaurants had effectively become another ordinary aspect of Philippine life (Business Asia

2000). In fact, AC Nielsen (2004) reports that some 99% of contemporary Filipinos are regular fast food patrons, with the country ranking only behind Hong Kong and Malaysia, and well above the U.S., as the top global market for this type of fare.

The rise of a new middle class has created conditions such that Filipino households now have more discretionary income and less time for preparing home-cooked meals as more women join the workforce. Domestic and foreign fast food companies have responded to this shifting demographic milieu by expanding their presence in Philippine towns and cities. At last estimate, there were over 3,000 quick-service eateries operating nationwide. In many ways, this proliferation can be viewed as a direct response to the demand created by middle class families for pre-cooked meals that are convenient, affordable, and served in clean and vibrant surroundings.

Such critical developments raise some fundamental questions about the globalization of corporate fast food, in general, and its local manifestations within the Philippines. Namely, how did multinational fast food companies first penetrate the Philippine market in the 1980s and gradually spread throughout the islands over subsequent decades? Moreover, what role did local and transnational capital play in facilitating this advance? To answer such questions, it useful to consider the experiences of the country's two most popular and long running burger chains—global fast food powerhouse McDonald's and its homegrown facsimile Jollibee. The intense competition that defines relations between these top brands in many ways sets the tone for ongoing developments within the country's overall fast food scene.

Over the past four decades these stalwarts of the Philippines' chain restaurant landscape have vied for control of the appetites and patronage of local consumers with often varying, if sometimes genuinely surprising, results. To wit, the country remains one of the few territories where the Golden Arches do not dominate fast food retailing (Economist 2002). Given its dominance of most other foreign markets, McDonald's runner-up status in the Philippines represents something of an embarrassment for the company (Conde 2005).

Interestingly, much of Jollibee's recent success comes from emulating the innovative standards and techniques that McDonald's pioneered in the U.S. years ago. The similarities and discontinuities that characterize their individual paths to success in the islands are rooted in the entrepreneurial efforts of two different Chinese-Filipino families who have risen to national and international prominence via their respective corporate visions and particular business approaches to selling fast food.

As the first major restaurant chain to popularize Western fast food in the Philippines, McDonald's entry into local commerce came just as the Marcos regime's hold on power began to weaken. Despite the precarious state of the country's political economy during this time, corporate fast food continued to expand in both scope and variety in Metro-Manila and beyond during the 1980s. An important dynamic underlying this growth was the developing rivalry between global and local brands. The initial success of McDonald's in the early and mid-1980s was soon eclipsed by the emergence Jollibee, whose intimate understanding of traditional foodways helped generate significant consumer followings nationwide. Part of what makes the company's dominance so notable is that it runs counter to prevailing Filipino assumptions that American brands and products are inherently superior to their local equivalents (Matejowsky 2007:30).

Against this backdrop, the ongoing competition between McDonald's and upstart Jollibee can be considered from various perspectives. In the strictest sense possible, it can be approached as two restaurant chains locked in a heated rivalry to control the country's growing fast food market. At a deeper level, it can also be viewed as a story rife with various sociopolitical overtones that unavoidably conveys as much about the Philippines' complicated postcolonial relationship with the U.S. as it does the complex interplay between hegemonic and counterhegemonic processes within the global fast food arena.

Within this latter viewpoint, the McDonald's/Jollibee rivalry helps delineate various tensions and compatibilities informing contemporary Filipino foodways just as it reveals certain paradoxes at play within the prevailing affinity for American culture previously mentioned. So, while this intense battle for burger supremacy provides an important entry point for understanding the varied textures and tastes of the Philippines' fast food scene, it simultaneously offers a viable framework for appreciating much about contemporary Filipino life and national identity with regard to the United States.

## GOLDEN ARCHES FILIPINO

The Golden Arches first appeared in the Philippines in 1981 when the country's inaugural restaurant was opened in Metro-Manila. Observing laws prohibiting majority foreign ownership, fast food multinationals like McDonald's were compelled to partner with indigenous firms to launch their brands locally. McGeorge Food Industries, a company headed by Chinese-Filipino retail magnate George Yang (b. 1939), secured the master franchise from McDonald's International. This licensing agreement gave Yang exclusive rights to operate McDonald's restaurants nationwide. In this way, Filipino companies like McGeorge gained the privileged use of iconic global brands and increased logistical know-how about fast food operations from their Western partners. In return, transnational chains secured footholds in previously untapped markets without assuming the associated risks of complete capitalization.

In the decades since it first entered the Philippine market, McDonald's has grown to around 375 outlets nationwide. While the majority of these eateries are managed and run by the company, close to 150 currently operate as local franchises. For those Filipino entrepreneurs with sufficient drive and capital, securing a 10-year franchise agreement with the Golden Arches typically goes for ₱30–50 million (U.S. $636,000–1 million) depending on the size, location, and equipment specifications. This working arrangement with McDonald's gives individual franchisees various kitchen and restaurant equipment including cash registers, signage, décor, air conditioning units, and emergency generators, it also plugs them into a network of other franchise owner-operators who provide advice and support to ensure the brand's success nationwide.

If there is any drawback to partnering with the Golden Arches in this capacity it may involve the rigidity to which franchisees are subjected in terms of daily operations. The company expects its franchise holders to follow a very detailed script when it comes to running their restaurants, leaving little opportunity for individual initiative or innovation.

In many ways, McDonald's expansion across the Philippines since the 1980s reflects both the popularization of corporate fast food among Filipinos and an ongoing transformation of local foodways and diets. The company has not only played a pivotal role in shaping the contours of fast food operations throughout the islands, it has also informed all manner of retail experience for Filipinos largely unacquainted with prompt, friendly, and highly scripted customer service.

Generations of Filipinos have frequented the Golden Arches over the years, developing a long-standing familiarity with the brand that is affectionately known locally by its abbreviated nickname "McDo." Just as the commercials and catchphrases associated with McDonald's have become an enduring aspect of Filipino popular culture, so too has its operations and menu items set a standard for other fast food companies to effectively measure themselves. The chain's almost outsized influence over contemporary life in the Philippines is something that could not have occurred without one man's visionary leadership.

## McGEORGE YANG

In December 2011, the *Philippine Star*, a national newspaper with a daily circulation of some 420,000 editions, ran a multipage color spread for their Sunday issue on George Yang, the celebrated company face of McDonald's in the Philippines (Sering 2011). The articles and interviews included in the extensive profile are written mostly by journalist and magazine editor Tara

Sering for an as-yet-unpublished biography on the Chinese-Filipino fast food magnate.

As a public figure, Yang is an ideal candidate for such an in-depth overview since for over three decades he has embodied a spirit of entrepreneurship that many Filipinos recognize as a bootstrapping success story. Besides running the Golden Arches operations all these years, he also holds stakes in a variety of real estate and commercial investments including the licensing rights for Disney and Marvel characters in the Philippines. A dedicated family man and trained singer of opera and traditional Filipino ballads with a string of albums and live performances under his belt, Yang is also involved with various McDonald's-affiliated charities charitable pursuits such as the Ronald McDonald House and Bright Minds Read, a school program that promotes storytelling and childhood literacy.

Composed not so much as hagiography of Yang but more as a detailed chronicle of his notable rise to prominence in the country's fast food scene and wider business community, the various accounts contained in the *Star* piece make public for the first time new levels of insight into his professional background, current family life, and ongoing charitable work. If anything, this mainstream coverage helps fill in some important gaps about how Yang got his start in the chain restaurant industry, secured the national McDonald's franchise for the Philippines, and ultimately elevated the Golden Arches to a position of national prestige second only to Jollibee within the nation's highly competitive fast food sector.

Details about Yang's family background are somewhat sparse in the *Philippine Star* feature beyond the fact that his entrepreneurial roots can be traced back to his paternal grandfather, Yang Wen Ying, and to a less degree his father, Yang Ing Kuong, both of whom found success in the Philippines' insurance sector in the 1950s and 1960s (Flores 2011). In fact, Yang's grandfather, an immigrant from mainland China, was able to start his own agency in the 1950s, United Insurance (later United Life), after years of working as an underwriter for another firm. Sering goes on to sketch out George Yang's educational and business pedigree prior to his ties with the McDonald's organization in the mid-1970s.

Despite some preliminary doubts about ever thriving in the Philippines' food industry, the younger Yang did hold aspirations of becoming a business owner of some sort, blazing a trail for himself by first completing an MBA from the prestigious Wharton School of Business at the University of Pennsylvania in 1964. Upon returning to the Philippines, he used some college connections to get hired by a local tobacco firm, Bataan Cigarettes, as a marketing manager. Alongside promoting tobacco products, Yang's early professional career also entailed moonlighting with various other jobs including selling insurance, peddling imported cosmetics, and teaching finance management and marketing at his undergraduate alma mater De La Salle University in Metro-Manila. Yang further expanded his business portfolio by developing a cigarette filter called Tar-Off and financially backing an upscale jewelry enterprise overseen by his equally industrious wife, Kristine (Sering 2011).

In a roundabout way, these diverse pursuits seemingly prepared Yang for something more ambitious in scale. Although he never actually patronized a McDonald's restaurant during his time in the United States (Flores 2011), like many Filipinos in the 1970s Yang was aware of the Golden Arches' considerable success in North America and increasingly overseas. Favorable coverage in the international business press about the chain reinforced such prevailing impressions. In 1974, after researching McDonald's operations in some detail, Yang contacted the company headquarters in Oakville, Illinois, with inquiries about opening restaurant branches in the Philippines.

At the time, McDonald's expressed little interest in gaining a foothold in this part of Southeast Asia. Despite an increasingly ripe climate for U.S. chain restaurants in the Philippines given the considerable imprint of American culture on Filipino lifeways over recent decades, the company remained largely unswayed by Yang's preliminary overtures of partnership. Far from discouraged by this initial rebuff, Yang began actively courting McDonald's executives by sending them both newspaper clippings about the Philippines and the occasional letter of good wishes in the hopes that they would not forget his keen interest in the company.

Yang's continuous outreach to McDonald's had the aggregate effect of convincing U.S. executives to rethink their initial indifference toward the Philippines. His efforts were so persuasive, in fact, that a team of company representatives travelled to the archipelago in 1976 to evaluate the feasibility of entering the Philippine market with Yang or possibly some other local partner. Since Yang was one of several potential franchisees vying for the opportunity to work with McDonald's, he had to find a way to effectively distinguish himself from his various more well-heeled rivals. As he told Sering, "The pitch was me," he explains. "I told them that if they wanted a long term partner, a partner who was going to roll up his sleeves and do the work, I was the one they were looking for. I told them this straight and was honest about who I was and what I was capable of" (Sering 2011).

While such sentiments, alongside the sterling business reputations of Yang and his family, helped ultimately sway McDonald's and their plans for the Philippines, it would be several years before the company actually established a market presence on the islands. Never one to sit by idly and allow external circumstances dictate his next move, Yang used this period of uncertainty to his distinct advantage.

Yang took the unusual step of voluntarily moving to nearby Hong Kong to better acquaint himself with the nuts and bolts of the fast food trade.

Specifically, he made arrangements with a business associate who held the McDonald's master franchise for the then-British territory to learn the operational aspects of running a company restaurant from the ground up. Yang temporarily relocated for several months with his 15-year-old son and future McGeorge CEO, Kenneth, to work as uniformed crewmembers at a McDonald's located in the city's bustling Kowloon district, performing a variety of tasks including cleaning toilets, swabbing floors, preparing burgers, and working the registers. Rising early and leaving late, father and son gained invaluable insights into running a successful McDonald's restaurant. More significantly, their immersive experience on the frontlines of McDonald's overseas operations reaffirmed Yang's determination to partner with the Golden Arches and make their prospective Philippines' venture a resounding success.

Such initiative on Yang's part apparently helped reinvigorate McDonald's long-gestating plans for the Philippines. Besides placing him in a much more positive light among chain executives, this kind of resourcefulness gave him an advantage over other would-be franchisees because Yang now had a decidedly more holistic understanding of how McDonald's operations actually worked. So, after a nearly four-year delay, the Golden Arches finally dispatched a team of company representatives to the islands in late 1980s with the news that Yang had edged out the competition to secure the Philippines' national franchise.

With little time to waste, Yang began taking steps to establish the country's first McDonald's in Metro-Manila's University Belt for the following year. More than anything else, he concentrated on creating a highly capable crew of managers to oversee all aspects of restaurant operations. With competitive wages and respectable compensation packages, Yang was able to attract and maintain an effective management team that has remained more or less intact throughout his tenure.

When reflecting back on the launch of the Philippines' first McDonald's eatery over 30 years later, Yang states "People were lining up, waiting to come in. So many people knew of the brand. We had to close the door to keep more people from coming into the store; otherwise it would just burst. It was very satisfying because all the time, hard work and efforts to get to that point" (Sering 2011). On the heels of this debut restaurant outlet, a second McDonald's branch was opened in Metro-Manila's tourist district, Cubao. Dozens of more eateries were to follow over the next decade both across the city and in communities throughout the main Philippine island of Luzon. It would not be until 1992 that McDonald's finally established a presence in a few major cities in the southern islands of the Visayas and Mindanao.

The chain's preliminary success in the Philippines rested largely on introducing Filipinos to those enduring aspects of fast food's international appeal, including a core menu of popular burgers and side items, quick and responsive customer service, and a family-friendly atmosphere. Even with such achievements, the country's fast food landscape did not remain static during McDonald's initial ascent. If anything, it became increasingly competitive as several new national and international brands commenced operations countrywide.

The Golden Arches recognized the necessity of adapting to these changing market conditions lest the company begin losing significant ground. To sustain its initial momentum and shore up its early position as industry bellwether amid an increasingly crowded chain restaurant scene, the ever resourceful Yang began looking for ways to innovate McDonald's standard quick-service format. Over the years his efforts at product improvement and restaurant efficiency have produced some notable results both in terms of menu offerings and customer service at the Golden Arches.

The challenges confronting Yang and McDonald's in terms of attracting and sustaining a viable consumer base amid a diversifying fast food landscape cannot be underestimated. By the mid-1980s, as the competition between national and transnational fast food intensified, many global chains like McDonald's began altering their operations to better conform to local tastes and customs. Although quick-service favorites like hamburgers and French fries were largely identical to those sold at U.S. restaurants, Philippine affiliates began incorporating new ingredients and selections to their core stationary menus.

These alterations typically entailed some kind of flavor sweetening or serving portions of steamed rice alongside certain entrées. Such retooling efforts were generally viewed as important steps toward the reassertion of global fast food chains as a dominant presence in local retailing. Over time, however, it became apparent that these changes were not quite enough to help McDonald's and other global chains alter the emerging consumer preference toward homegrown brands like Jollibee.

In terms of food, McGeorge developed various new products that better resonated with more traditional Filipino palates. In 1986, McSpaghetti (pasta noodles with sweet tomato sauce and chopped frankfurter bits) was introduced to restaurant menu boards across the islands as an alternative to the perennial standbys of Big Macs, Quarter Pounders, and French fries. This popular fare was followed two years later by the Chicken McDo (fried chicken, steamed rice, and gravy), a more sumptuous meal selection that features steamed rice as a side item (Ritzer 2000:173). In 1993, a distinctively Filipino take on the standard McDonald's hamburger was launched. Known as the Burger McDo, this sandwich has a much more understated flavor that jibed well with Filipinos' general aversion to sharp and tangy ingredients (Sering 2011). Other snacks and meals created for McDonald's Philippine market during this period include the popular mango shake and breakfast favorite, longganisa with rice.

Apart from these locally inspired dishes, McDonald's also innovated other aspects of its restaurant operations. In 1982, the company opened the Philippines' first drive-thru restaurant in the affluent Manila suburb of Greenhills. This service lane would later become an increasingly pervasive feature of McDonald's restaurants as McGeorge established more and more free-standing outlets along high-traffic thoroughfares across the islands.

Other innovations included the introduction of on-site playgrounds, kids' birthday parties, standalone Dessert Centers (kiosks that sell ice cream and other desserts in mall parking lots and other public places), and a phone-based food delivery service called 8-MCDO that was launched by the Golden Arches in 2002. Given its success with fast food patrons, this latter offering has been expanded to include new ways for McDonald's to supply its customers with take-out cuisine such as the 24/7 McDelivery service, which makes ordering available to diners at all times, as well as more recent web-based delivery system (Sering 2011). Walk-up windows are a more recent improvement now found at many urban McDonald's. This feature allows diners to bypass a restaurant's traditional customer queue and place take-out orders through a sliding glass window that faces the sidewalk under a protective awning.

To publicize McDonald's products and services, the company has engaged in many memorable television, web, and print advertising campaigns that have variously captured the imaginations of Filipino audiences. These promotional initiatives often feature celebrity endorsers like Filipina actress/singer/talk show host Sharon Cuenta and international boxing phenomenon Manny Pacquiao. Not so different from McDonald's commercials in other parts of the globe in terms of tone and product emphasis, such local marketing efforts typically have storylines to which everyday Filipino families and children can relate. In some cases, they even highlight timely social issues that confront millions of households nationwide. For example, in the 1990s, a few commercials starring Cuenta centered on the familiar domestic situation of parents or close kin working abroad as OCWs. Beyond such narrative elements, these adverts also feature catchy jingles or showcase company catchphrases such as *Ulitin Ang Sarap!* (Repeat the deliciousness!) and *Love ko 'to* (I'm lovin' it).

McDonald's Philippines operations continue to carve out a viable presence in communities across the Visayas, Luzon, and Mindanao despite being eclipsed by domestic competitor Jollibee in terms of sales and popularity beginning in the mid-1980s. Even though it has now lagged behind its main rival for some three decades among the country's burger buying public, McGeorge is still well regarded by its McDonald's counterparts in the United States and elsewhere. In fact, Yang and company have won the McDonald's

International Award for Excellence in profitability and value in both 1996 and 1997.

Beginning in the early 2000s, the senior Yang has ceded more and more of his leadership responsibilities with McDonald's to his son Kenneth and other children working within the organization. Despite such gradual abdication, he still remains focused on the company expansion and innovation, telling Sering (2011) that he hopes to expand the number of Golden Arches in the Philippines to 500 by 2015.

With the benefit of hindsight, it is easy to see just what an impact McDonald's and George Yang have had on the Philippines's current fast food scene. Without his tenacity and entrepreneurial drive, it remains uncertain as to when the Golden Arches would have finally entered the Philippine market much less how the country's chain restaurant landscape would ultimately develop. Without the corporate rivalry between McDonald's and Jollibee that continues to define so much of the prevailing manifestations of fast food production and consumption nationwide, it is unclear just how motivated either firm would be in offering customers new and innovative dining experiences.

While McDonald's inability to sufficiently reassert its market dominance within the Philippines and thereby transcend its longtime runner-up position to Jollibee may still aggravate corporate executives in the United States and elsewhere, there is doubtless something to be said about the brand's undeniable resilience and staying power. Quite simply, without the innovations developed by the Golden Arches over the years, it is entirely probable that Jollibee and other domestic quick-service eateries would not have achieved their current level of success and popularity among Filipino consumers.

## THE GLOBAL RISE AND CONTINUED DOMINANCE OF JOLLIBEE

Perhaps more so than the press coverage directed at McDonald's and its decades-long presence in the Philippines, a considerable amount of ink has been spilled over the years in various magazines, newspapers, and web publications on Jollibee and its remarkable ascendancy to the top of the country's chain restaurant scene (Conde 2005; Cuevas 2007; De Leon 2013; Economist 2002; Stein 2007). Whether presented in national or international media, these accounts rarely neglect highlighting the company's decades-longs lead over the Golden Arches in local fast food retailing. In this way, it bears reiterating that, while McDonald's has historically dominated the chain restaurant landscape in whatever global market it has launched operations, the Philippines remains one of the few countries where an indigenous brand holds the distinction of most popular quick-service burger joint (Economist 2002).

For non-Filipinos, such glowing reportage about Jollibee can at times come across as overly congratulatory, especially when these sentiments are tailored toward Filipino audiences whether living at home or abroad (De Leon 2013). Understandably, there is probably something journalistically irresistible about a storyline featuring a homegrown restaurant operation emerging seemingly out of nowhere to compete against and eventually wrest away the title of the Philippines' favorite quick-service chain restaurant from the world's seminal fast food brand. Suffice it to say, the competition between McDonald's and Jollibee within the Philippines serves as an almost inescapable feature of the country's fast food scene.

## THE BEEKEEPER

Given such favorable media attention and widespread public support, it is perhaps unsurprising that Jollibee Food Corporation's meteoric rise to the top of the Philippines' fast food industry now approaches the stuff of national legend. The chain restaurant giant, founded by ethnic Chinese entrepreneur Tony Tan Caktiong and his brothers some four decades ago, has become all but enshrined in Filipino popular culture in a way that few other native corporations can effectively approach (De Leon 2013).

The company has cultivated a substantial consumer base that responds to its corporate brand image almost as much as it does the restaurant's distinctive menu items. Such positive responses have translated into an ongoing patronage of repeat customers that seemingly transcends generations. In ways that reflect Filipinos' intense focus on extended kin relations, it is not uncommon to see tables of parents, grandparents, and children dining alongside other patrons eating alone or in groups. This loyal consumer following has led to considerable earnings for Jollibee over the years.

These profits have, in turn, helped Jollibee consolidate its market supremacy with the purchase of several local and foreign fast food chains including Greenwich Pizza, Red Ribbon (bakeshop), Mang Inasal (chicken and barbecue), Burger King Philippines, and Chowking in the early and mid-2000s. More recently, the company has acquired significant shares in fast casual restaurants operating in the United States such as Smashburger (hamburgers and fries) and Jinja Bar and Bistro (Pacific and Asian fusion) and a few quick-service noodle chains located in mainland Asia including China's Hong Zhuang Yun (congee) and San Pin Wang (beef noodles) as well as Vietnam's Pho 24 (noodles). When its network of approximately 3,000 (630 are abroad) branches and franchises of the various brands operating under the Jollibee Food Corporation umbrella are taken into consideration together, it is not surprising that Jollibee now ranks as Asia's largest restaurant company.

More than half of Jollibee and its subsidiary restaurants currently operate as franchises. In fact, this approach to licensing the company brand and ancillary services to local partners has proven one of the key elements in Jollibee's ongoing success. Like other global fast food chains, Jollibee strives to find entrepreneurially oriented individuals and firms to work with at the community level. As one representative stated in 1997, "We seek individuals with a spirit of enterprise who will commit to building the Jollibee business. Experience in hotel and restaurant is not a must. They should have good business background with good people handling skills and (be) willing to spend time and effort to the restaurant business" (Paradeza 1997).

This approach to restaurant operations clearly helps minimize risk for the company. At the same time, it offers a reputable brand that customers both recognize and appreciate as well as a proven storehouse of operational knowledge that franchisees can readily draw upon. Although anyone can technically apply to run a Jollibee or one of its sister eateries as a franchise, a rigorous screening process tends to weed out all but the most qualified of applicants. Prospective franchisees who want to are required to assemble a detailed submission packet that includes materials such as a completed application form, letter of intent, vicinity map of the proposed site, and comprehensive résumé. Potential partners then have to wait a month or two for the company's decision.

The franchise grant for prospective restaurateurs is typically for a 10-year period and runs upwards of ₱25–35 million (U.S. $530,00–741,000) for mall or fast food center locations. The price tag for free-standing outlets—that is, those constructed on a vacant lot—is even more. If successful in their franchise bids, new restaurant operators are expected to adhere to the specific operating procedures established by Jollibee in order to ensure consistency and uniformity to menu and dining experience. Again this sort of top-down rigidity is something perfected by McDonald's and savvily replicated by Jollibee.

The eponymous Jollibee restaurant chain currently maintains a substantial presence in the Philippines with some 900 outlets operating nationwide. There are also about 135 locations in other parts of the world on three different continents. Jollibee eateries can be found in Vietnam, Indonesia, Hong Kong, Brunei, Dubai, United Arab Emirates, Great Britain, Italy, and Canada, as well as in major U.S. cities such as Las Vegas, Los Angeles, San Francisco, San Diego, New York, Chicago, and Jersey City (Economist 2016).

This number is up from 2007 when just over 575 outlets were in operation domestically and abroad. Not coincidently most of these overseas Jollibee locations have opened in countries and regions with an already sizable community of Filipino expatriates and temporary workers. Filipino-Americans, balikbayans, and OCWs represent a significant segment of the company's overseas market. The availability of familiar menu items and restaurant surroundings doubtless offers a welcome opportunity to experience some of the comforts of home, however modest, while living or working abroad. A domestic worker living in Hong Kong alludes to this sentiment saying, "All Filipinos love Jollibee because we feel like we are at home" (De Leon 2013).

Obviously the company's commanding presence over fast food in the Philippines owes much to the business savvy and entrepreneurial resolve of Tan Caktiong. Born in 1934 and earning a Civil Engineering degree from the University of Santo Tomas, Tan Caktiong did not seem particularly destined for his future role as a fast food mogul. His father, Tan Eng Lan, worked for a time as a restaurant chef in the southern city of Davao before a family relocation to Metro-Manila where he found work as a chef at a Buddhist monastery. As family lore has it, Tony had a very discerning palate when it comes to taste and ingredients. Unlike his siblings, he only ate the most simply prepared of dishes and seemed more interested in engineering (De Leon 2013).

Today, Tony Tan Caktiong stands as one of the wealthiest living Filipinos with a net worth of just over one billion U.S. dollars (Forbes 2015). Like his rival George Yang, Tony Tan Caktiong values the abilities of his children and extended kin when it comes to running aspects of the Jollibee brand. The vast global fast food empire he currently oversees in many ways belies its rather humble origins in the 1970s. His ability to transform Jollibee into an iconic global chain holds particular resonance within the Philippines' wider business community in the sense that it vividly illustrates what can happen when the right kind of entrepreneur capitalizes on favorable market conditions within an emerging consumer sector.

## FROM ICE CREAM TO HAMBURGERS

Jollibee traces its roots back to a pair of neighborhood ice cream parlors located in Cubao and Quiapo, two of Metro-Manila's oldest and densely populated urban districts. While still a chemistry student, Tan Caktiong visited a Magnolia Ice Cream production facility with his future wife Grace. Impressed with what they saw, the couple seized a franchise opportunity with the popular frozen dessert brand, launching two company-affiliated branch locations in 1975. These original family-run enterprises operated for a few years as ice cream and soda fountain shops before eventually shifting focus to hamburgers and French fries after these one-time side items proved more popular with customers than the signature dairy products.

Similarly, the chain's name went through several iterations until Tan Caktiong and his marketing consultant Manuel Lumba finally settled on the now iconic "Jollibee." Early on, the restaurant was known as "Jolibe" and,

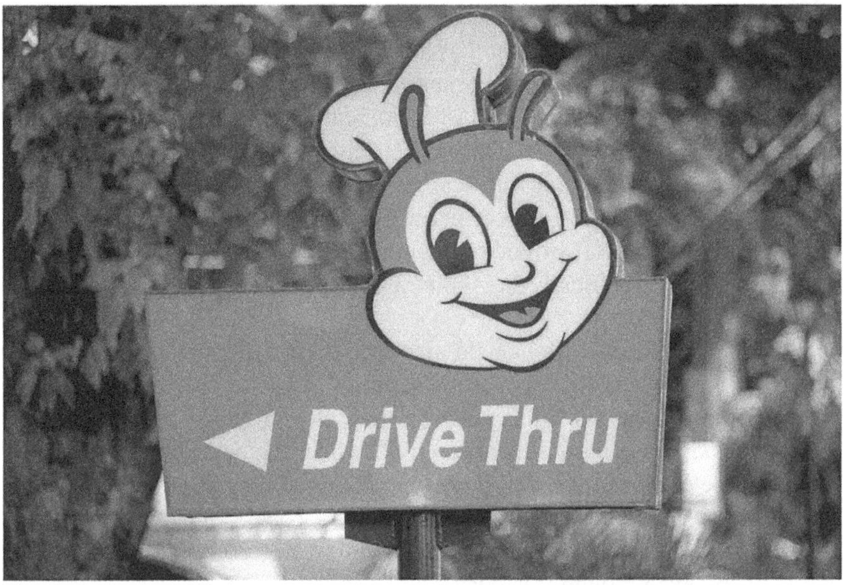


**Figure 2.1 Jollibee drive through sign, Philippines.** © iStock.com/holgs.

then, "Jolibee" before the insertion of an additional "L." As Lumba explains "Among Filipinos, "Jolibe" didn't ring a bell. But without throwing it away, we added another "L" and an "E" to now mean "jolly bee." While it was wrongly spelled, I chose to keep it, and now we had a memorable name" (Imbong 2015). In no small way, this early ability to shrewdly anticipate and react to consumer demand and sentiment has expanded significantly over the years, serving the company quite well in various areas of operation.

Part of Jollibee's continuing success in the Philippines and elsewhere rests in its tactic of adopting and refining those techniques and practices developed by other leading companies. Service industry innovations from the likes of the Walt Disney Company and various global air carriers have been integrated into Jollibee operations over the years to improve the restaurant experience for consumers (De Leon 2013). Probably more relevant is the adoption of those operational aspects developed by rival fast food firms such as the Golden Arches.

Early on, the Tan Caktiongs paid careful attention to McDonald's overseas ventures, noting what developments proved effective for the company and what efforts did not. Such observations helped establish the working model for Jollibee restaurant operations for years to come. From a nearly duplicate color scheme that emphasizes red and other warmish colors to a food preparation system that is nearly interchangeable with the one originated by

McDonald's decades before, Jollibee has made no real secret of replicating those aspects of the global giant that have achieved positive results.

Jollibee's locally ubiquitous corporate mascot—a smiling cartoon bee in a chef's hat—was introduced in 1980 and bears a more than passing resemblance to the iconic Ronald McDonald. His distinctive image crops up in various places around Philippine cityscapes including jeepney stops, schoolyard murals, and town plazas. Like the perpetually upbeat clown, the giant cherubic bee sports a colorful striped outfit, surrounding himself with a collection of fast food–inspired friends that prominently appear in chain advertising and promotional items.

Besides such Ronald McDonald similarities, the restaurant's bee mascot also features its share of Disneyesque qualities (Imbong 2015). These appear most prominently in his Mickey Mouse-like gloved hands and exaggerated puffy cheeks. These more superficial traits aside, the decision to have a bee represent the company is based on certain core qualities that everyday working Filipinos share with these social insects. As Tony Tan Caktiong tells the Economist (2002), "the bee hops around and produces sweet things for life, and is happy even though it is busy."

If anything, the bee reflects what Tan Caktiong sees as the unwavering spirit of ordinary Filipinos who confront life's challenges with a perennially optimistic and sometimes playful outlook. Such notions are also reaffirmed in how staffers greet customers and each other. As a matter of deference, crew members are required to use the traditional honorifics of "sir" and "mom" in all interactions. This practice plays well in the Philippines, a society where respect for one's elders remains a deeply ingrained aspect of social life (Economist 2002).

The child-centric approach seemingly perfected by McDonald's also extends to other facets of Jollibee restaurant operations including the presence of indoor playgrounds, the addition of toys and tie-in products from the latest summer blockbuster in various kids' meal offerings, and the availability of store space and resources for birthday and community celebrations. As will be explored in more ethnographic detail in subsequent chapters, this marketing orientation toward families with young children has paid real dividends for Jollibee and its fast food rivals.

No less significant as considerations about family and children, Jollibee also continues to pursue an aggressive expansion and marketing plan that makes comparable efforts by McDonald's in the Philippines appear relatively cautious. The Tan Caktiongs reportedly spent their first few years' profits on restaurant advertising in an effort to hype public interest in the chain. For some time, they have similarly followed an ambitious two-to-one development strategy, establishing two Jollibee outlets for every restaurant operated by the Golden Arches (Quimpo-Espino 2004).

As things currently stand, there are almost two and a half times as many eponymous Jollibee eateries in the Philippines compared to those affiliated with McDonald's. Such avid dedication to growth and innovation has enhanced public perception of Jollibee's dynamic productivity compared to that of McDonald's and other national and international fast food operators. If truth be told, once the prevailing consensus about Jollibee's ascendancy took root in the public consciousness, the Golden Arches came to be viewed as nothing so much as the country's perennial second-place fast food brand.

No less integral to Jollibee's ascendancy is the firm's deep grasp of the Filipino palate. If anything, this keen understanding of what Filipinos find flavorsome and unsavory has continually worked to the company's advantage. More so than its competitors, Jollibee has been able to develop products that appeal to local tastes. These include favorites such as serving a wide selection of Filipino favorites like Chickenjoy (fried chicken and rice), Champs (large hamburgers), Yums! (small hamburgers), Jolly Spaghetti (Bolognese mixed with sliced red frankfurters), Shanghai Rolls (fried spring rolls), Jolly Dogs (red hotdogs with white cheese and mayonnaise), Burger Steaks (hamburger patties smothered in mushrooms and gravy), Amazing Aloha Champ Burger (bacon-cheeseburger with mayonnaise and sliced pineapple), and Palabok Fiesta (traditional Filipino pasta slathered with a special pork-shrimp sauce, garlic, eggs, and meat).

In order to meet the logistical demands of a dining public that continuously craves the products of its flagship chain and various subsidiaries, Jollibee maintains the Zenith Food Corp. Commissary, a six-hectare industrial facility in Central Luzon that employs approximately 500 personnel working round the clock over three shifts, seven days a week. Each day the commissary processes some 20 tons of Chickenjoy, 40 tons of ground beef patties, 56 tons of sauce (mostly spaghetti), 200,000 pies, and 23 tons of hotdogs, all of which are shipped to the hundreds of branches and outlets located around the islands. Based on demand projections from individual stores, supply planning begins near two months before delivery (Philippine Star 2008).

At the commissary, various production lines are continuously operational. Two of the most active are dedicated to the production of beef patties and hamburger buns (Philippine Star 2008). Burger meat comes from various global sources including suppliers based out of Brazil, New Zealand, and Australia. Upon delivery, this high-grade beef undergoes all type of processing. It is ground, marinated, and formed into patties before finally being frozen into individual units.

Meat safety and freshness is ensured through the application of blast freezers and metal detectors. Similarly, numerous steps are followed in the production of hamburger buns. In fact, by the time they are packaged for shipping, these baked goods have gone through nearly two kilometers of

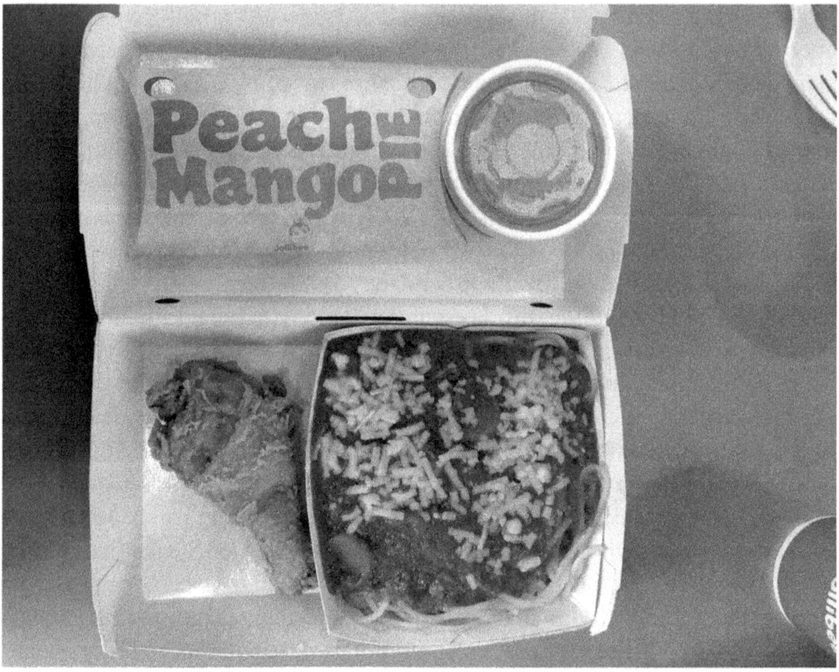


**Figure 2.2 Jollibee Chickenjoy and Spaghetti, Jacksonville, Florida August 2017.** Photo taken by Lorena Parker Matejowsky.

conveyor belts (Philippine Star 2008). Hotdogs, meatballs, spiced ham, and some sauces are created in a meat production line while the chickens for the best-selling Chickenjoy are dressed, marinated, frozen, and packaged for shipment.

Most of these Jollibee menu items are notably sweeter and juicier than the food served at McDonald's and other Western fast food outlets (Economist 2002). The company utilizes a research and development team to ensure consistency across all product lines (Philippine Star 2008). When weighed against the sweet succulence of Jollibee's signature bill of fare, McDonald's cuisine comes across as relatively dry, bland, and sometimes sour. Thus, whereas McDonald's serves tomato ketchup and dill pickles with its hamburgers, Jollibee opts for the more saccharine tastes of banana ketchup and sweet pickles. For dessert, McDonald's offers fried apple pies and chocolate sundaes, while Jollibee counters with the locally popular fried peach mango pies and mango shakes. For many everyday Filipinos, these differences in flavor and ingredients can become the decisive factor if given a choice between dining at the Golden Arches or taking a meal at Jollibee.

Indeed, such taste preferences were expressed to me directly in July 2005 from Hazel, the 20-year-old niece of the woman in whose household I lived as a boarder in Dagupan City over the years. When I asked her if she prefers the menu of Jollibee over McDonald's, she replied "The food at Jollibee is more Filipino. Sweeter. The French fries at McDo are too salty." Building off her comments my research assistant, Mario, added "McDo's food is tomato-based. Jollibee is sweeter." Taken as a whole, Jollibee's ability to satisfy Filipino appetites, coupled with an efficient service model, has proven a winning formula for the company.

Thus, thanks to an aggressive marketing plan and innovative menu, Jollibee has remained the top fast food player in the Philippines since 1984. According to the Economist (2016) Jollibee's system-wide sales—which gauge all the sales to consumers and franchised stores—and net profits rose by around 70 percent to ₱118 billion ($2.5 billion) and ₱5.4 billion, respectively. Forecasts for continued success remain mostly positive as the Philippine economy has benefitted over recent years from the outsourcing of call-centers and other business operations from the Global North to the point where overall consumer spending can now support a robust fast food scene. Such developments, alongside a strong upper and middle management, bode well for future growth as Jollibee strives to make further inroads into lucrative foreign markets like the United States and China with its namesake restaurant and various subsidiary chains.

## FAST FOOD PATRIOTISM?

Obviously, a number of affiliated factors contribute to Jollibee's ongoing market supremacy in the Philippines. Matters related to marketing, taste, geographical availability, and entrepreneurial initiative all help shape the composition of the country's fast food landscape. Yet, part of Jollibee's enduring appeal among Filipinos both at home and abroad is that its decades-long lead over the Golden Arches easily translates into a kind of narrative framework whereby David overcomes Goliath with seemingly minimal effort. The fact that a local fast food start-up essentially comes out of nowhere to supplant a formidable and highly capitalized global brand in the nation's burgeoning chain restaurant sector resonates in a highly effective way (Economist 2002). While the veracity of this corporate mythology surely glosses over conflicting and incongruous story elements, it nevertheless captures the rivalry between Jollibee and McDonald's essence in most key respects.

In this way, the deep brand loyalty enjoyed by Jollibee also reflects underlying political and/or patriotic dimensions that frequently remain under-acknowledged by outside observers. Reaffirming what was stated in chapter 1, multinational fast food is frequently viewed as the cutting edge of an emerging global consumer culture, one that works to undermine local traditions and institutions to the point that societies worldwide become increasingly homogenous and deterritorialized (Friedman 1999:21; Ritzer 2004: 175–176). Yet, as noted throughout this and other works, this scenario is only true up to a point. The rapid proliferation of chain eateries across global foodscapes over the past four decades also creates spaces for the articulation of nationalist sentiments and expressions of locality that are often empowering if not openly counterhegemonic in nature.

While sociologist Uri Ram does (2004) observe a particular type of global homogenization occurring at the structural-institutional level as chain restaurants like KFC and McDonald's become more and more entrenched in non-Western milieus, the impact of this process is much less penetrative than most initially perceive. Given the highly regimented uniformity in the Fordist preparation style of corporate fast food, alongside a basic consistency in its restaurant design and signage, it seems all but inevitable that a discernible kind of sameness begins to emerge.

Yet, just as these standardized elements prove quite adaptable to different cultural contexts over time, they also tend to obscure the various heterogeneities that now characterize local fast food scenes worldwide. Doubtless, as American-style fast food continues to gain momentum in diverse foreign markets, these operations become more and more decoupled from their primary origins in the United States and Europe. So much so, in fact, that a McDonald's operating in today's Philippines features practices and traits that appear largely unfamiliar to its Western diners.

Indeed, it is at an expressive-symbolic level where homegrown fast food producers and consumers engage this versatile dining format with a considerable degree of agency and indigenization. Ram (2004) suggests that ideas of cuisine, flavor, and national/cultural identity have undergone their fair share of reconfiguration and reinvention as quick-service eateries take root globally. For example, he documents how the emergence of McDonald's in Israel in the 1990s not only revived consumer interest in gourmet falafels among local fast casual diners but also drew notable political distinctions between the Golden Arches and indigenous brands. Such developments are notably evident in the long-standing rivalry between McDonald's and Jollibee in the Philippines.

Within this expressive-symbolic stratum, it is probably not surprising that choices about where to dine and what to order can now reflect patriotic sentiments almost as much as they do feelings of brand allegiance. Local manifestations of corporate fast food have reinvigorated aspects of cultural, national, and class identity in various settings around the world (Wu 1997). In particular, restaurant preferences are beginning to reveal genuine, if sometimes subtle, expressions of postcolonial resistance against globalization and its ostensible homogenizing tendencies. The ambivalence that many in what was once called the Third World feel about outside corporate interests and their considerable sway over local life is increasingly apparent in consumer attitudes and predilections toward homegrown fast food companies like Jollibee (Stein 2007).

The considerable edge Jollibee enjoys over McDonald's in the Philippines is informed by certain political and nationalist connotations that in their own way probably say as much about everyday Filipinos and their complicated historical relationship with America as they do about how corporate fast food intersects with nearly all aspects of global modernity. Indeed, locals seem to readily embrace this most American way of dining formats while simultaneously applauding the fact that pioneering U.S. brands lag behind their homegrown counterparts. Such patriotic associations assume particular dimension in select company promotions, including the frequently asked questions section of Jollibee's corporate homepage where a series of queries are posed to company CEO Tony Tan Caktiong, including the following:

> What about [Jollibee] reshaping national values and orientation?
>
> TTC's [Tony Tan Caktiong's] Jollibee—its romping of McDonald's in the Philippines and entry into the latter's US turf (a reversal of trend)—makes one proud to be a Filipino. It makes one feel, indeed, the Filipino can.
>
> During the country's centennial celebration [1998], Jollibee launched a series of advertising campaigns centered on nationalism and respect for the Filipino flag. The series brought to the limelight Jollibee's strong national pride and faith in the Filipino. (Jollibee 2007)

This sort of patriotic messaging, coupled with the kinds of locally inspired fast food items and concentrated marketing efforts for which Jollibee is now known, has worked to define the company as a highly successful national brand that can outcompete more seasoned chains from the United States and elsewhere. As the case of Jollibee in the Philippines makes clear, industry giants such as McDonald's, KFC, and Pizza Hut have sometimes struggled to realign themselves in overseas markets as new domestic players exert more control over local eating habits (Stein 2007). With competition between national and transnational chains intensifying worldwide (Rai 2005), fast food consumption takes on added political dimension, especially in advanced developing countries.

Bearing in mind the historical roots of corporate fast food, ongoing chain rivalries, and sometimes under-articulated national and political sentiments maintained by local fast food diners, a relevant backdrop for a more detailed and reflexive account of quick-service eateries is effectively delineated. The next chapter builds off of these descriptions by narrowing ethnographic focus to the fast food scenes of two tertiary cities in the north-central Philippines: the aforementioned Dagupan City, Pangasinan and San Fernando City, La Union.

After providing basic demographic, geographical, and historical information for these neighboring communities, I will trace major commercial developments that have variously transformed both cities over the past three decades before shifting focus to the emergence of their respective fast food sectors. Interspersed among these descriptions are some of my own observations and experiences related to recent corporate fast food developments and restaurant operations in both cities. These more personal accounts are included primarily to enhance ethnographic granularity and provide readers a more on-the-ground perspective. Paying particular attention to the individuals and events that expedited the establishment or in some cases the failure of various national and international quick-service eateries at the community level beginning in the 1980s, this chapter offers dual accounts of how corporate chain restaurants penetrate local commerce in provincial areas, adding both depth and insight to prevailing notions about the hegemony of global fast food.

# Chapter 3

# A Tale of Two Local Fast Food Scenes

## *Corporate Fast Food in Dagupan City, Pangasinan and San Fernando City, La Union 1980s–2010s*

The success of national and international fast food chains in and around Metro-Manila beginning in the early 1980s revealed several important things. Not only did it show just how adaptable this dining format is across diverse cultural contexts, it also highlighted Filipinos' enduring openness to nearly all things American, including the production and marketing of corporate fast food (Matejowsky 2007). Perhaps most importantly to McDonald's, Jollibee, and other restaurant brands, it also demonstrated that Filipinos had cultivated a sufficient enough taste for this style of cuisine so that a loyal customer base nationwide was no longer viewed as an open question.

By all indications Filipinos loved their fast food whether it was served up as hamburgers, spaghetti, fried chicken, or French fries. So popular was this convenience fare, in fact, that restaurant companies started looking into smaller provincial markets as the logical next step in their expansion plans.

Such targeted growth and developments coincided with a reemergence of political and financial stability in the post-Marcos era (1986–1992). This general reduction in volatility both increased investor confidence in the Philippines and contributed to a burgeoning urban middle class looking to spend its newfound discretionary income on all sorts of Western-style consumer experiences. Even as significant socioeconomic disparities persisted across the Visayas, Mindanao, and Luzon during this time, the purchasing power of well-off and modestly affluent households reached a point where this sort of expansion was economically viable. Although the 1997 Asian financial crisis engendered a period of market instability whereby investor and consumer confidence declined precipitously, the country was able to weather such ill-effects and eventually resume mostly consistent economic growth over subsequent years.

Throughout the 1990s and beyond, both Jollibee and McDonald's remained at the forefront of such market penetration into the Philippine hinterland. Significantly, these rival firms were not alone in this regard as secondary brands and subsidiaries including Chowking, Greenwich Pizza, KFC, and others also worked to create a foothold, albeit less pronounced, away from the country's most populous urban center. Over time this slate of quick-service eateries would come to include Burger King, Pizza Hut, Kenny Rogers' Roasters, A&W, and several other global and homegrown chains.

While individual restaurant brands would strive to gain a competitive edge over their rivals within this increasingly crowded field, not all would achieve the same level of success. In fact, as will be touched upon later in this chapter when looking at Dagupan and San Fernando City specifically, some of these eateries would flourish while others would struggle to establish a local niche, eventually scaling down operations or going out of business entirely.

As the number of provincial towns and cities developing fast food scenes of their own increased during the 1980s and 1990s, so too did various shifts in local political economies began to emerge. Such changes were perhaps most vividly expressed within the street-level urban fabric of local built environments. Indeed, the often austere surroundings of downtown business districts suddenly appeared less drab with the appearance of new chain eateries sporting sleek signage and flashy consumer aesthetics. Enhancing this ongoing transformation in urban character was the addition of several modern supermarkets whose aisles teemed with all variety of manufactured goods and food items. These offerings, coupled with new amenities like automated checkout scanners and lanes, moved local food shopping and consumption in a decidedly more global direction. When considered altogether, the overall identity of provincial urban centers assumed a decidedly more cosmopolitan edge with area residents now able to partake in a global consumer culture that was previously not so readily accessible. Traveling to Metro-Manila, Cebu City, or some other major metropolitan center no longer represented the only real option for Filipinos looking to experience such American-style restaurants or shopping ventures.

For some provincial Filipinos, the encroachment of new ventures like corporate fast food into local commerce was even embraced as evidence that their hometowns were now outpacing the trade sectors of those neighboring communities still lacking viable fast food and retail scenes (Matejowsky 2006). Even if such sentiments were not entirely well-founded, they certainly did little to curb growing enthusiasm for the local availability of this style of dining and consumption. Fast food menu items and amenities soon provided a convenient, if even slightly more expensive, dining option for consumers increasingly on-the-go. This sort of ease and availability, coupled with an ongoing receptiveness to local variations of hamburgers, French fries, and other American-style cuisine among townsfolk, boded well for the future of

Jollibee, McDonald's, and their competitors beyond the primary market of Metro-Manila.

Yet, for all the seemingly positive outcomes and civic pride associated with the expansion of quick-service eateries and other modern food outlets into provincial towns and cities, their launch also proved problematic in that they sometimes aggravate lingering problems in urban life. For example, the arrival of new chain restaurants within often congested downtown settings did little to improve local traffic patterns. Almost immediately, the need for additional private vehicle parking and drop-off zones for passenger jeepneys to adequately accommodate this surge of customers was compounded. Additionally, these new operations also emerged as a discernible threat to existing mom-and-pop eateries whose traditional clientele were suddenly subject to the fresh allure of these state-of-the-art dining venues. Moreover, the arrival of eateries like McDonald's and Jollibee exacerbated perennial issues of littering within city centers. Corporate fast food's reliance on paper wrappers and other disposal food packaging and receptacles quickly came into evidence along urban, streets, sidewalks, and vacant areas.

Clearly, the proliferation of quick-service eateries in the Philippine hinterland throughout these years has added new wrinkles to local lifeways (Matejowsky 2007). In an effort to understand how the changes produced by corporate fast food's provincial growth played out at the community level, I turn attention to the respective experiences of Dagupan City, Pangasinan and San Fernando City, La Union. While the penetration of chain eateries into regional markets is often approached as a unidirectional process that leaves local interests effectively powerless to impede or arrest its unrelenting advance, such narratives do not always align with the experience of affected communities.

To create a more complete portrait of how American-style fast food companies extend their reach beyond major metropolitan centers and establish a viable presence at the municipal level in secondary and tertiary cities, it is important to consider the role of local capital in this process. As the forthcoming cases from Dagupan and San Fernando suggest, corporate fast food's encroachment into previously untapped provincial areas could not have occurred without the efforts of local entrepreneurs and enterprises. More specifically, the role of franchising, established political clout, and ethnic retail firms cannot be underestimated in this unfolding process.

## DAGUPAN CITY, PANGASINAN—HISTORY AND SOCIOECONOMIC STRUCTURE

Located some 220 kilometers north of Metro-Manila, Dagupan is a coastal city comprised of around 164,000 residents living in approximately 37,000 households spread across 31 municipal precincts. The municipality has long served as one of the north-central Philippines' most important and accessible commercial, financial, and educational centers with various provincial colleges and universities operating in and around its *población* (city center).

The history of Dagupan stretches back to pre-Hispanic times. Prior to the arrival of Augustinian monks to the region in 1590, indigenous groups had already established a presence along the common delta formed by the Agno, Toboy, Bued-Angalacan, and Pantal Rivers. These native inhabitants exploited the fertile conditions of this estuarial environment, subsisting primarily through fishing and rice cultivation. Numerous inland waterways and accessibility to the Lingayen Gulf established the community as an important center of coastal life. Early Dagupeños maintained trade ties with tribal populations living in interior Pangasinan as well as seafaring Chinese merchants on their occasional sojourns to northern Luzon (Basa 1997).

The indigenous settlement predating modern Dagupan was formally organized into a town by the Spanish in 1643. A native uprising in 1660 destroyed much of the colonial infrastructure which, in turn, lead to the community's being named *Nandaragupan* (Vistro and Reyes 2005). Roughly translated as "where once stood the commercial center," this title remained prominent for nearly a century before the more simplified name "Dagupan" was adopted in the late eighteenth century (Active Research Center 1994:38). For most of its colonial experience the town served as a rice farming and coastal fishing village. As technological advances took root in this part of the provincial Philippines throughout the 1800s, Dagupan began to evolve into a thriving commercial center. In 1855, the nearby port of Sual opened to international trade. This helped elevate Dagupan's position as an important link in the maritime traffic of commodities from the Illocos region to the north, via Sual, to Manila. Soon, Dagupan started outpacing neighboring communities as northern Luzon's principal entrepôt.

Local trade activity in 1885 is described as follows:

> With the arrival of the northeast monsoon mercantile enterprises begin. The port of Dagupan becomes filled with ponties [*sic*] and other craft serving coastal traffic, which carry goods to Manila. In this period there is much movement up until . . . . June and July when the wet season commences and traffic is paralyzed, and the boats depart, seeking shelter until the return of the fair season. (Carrozal 1886, quoted in Trager 1988:26)

As Dagupan's economic vitality became more pronounced in the mid- and late nineteenth century, so too did the presence of foreign-owned commercial ventures. Several enterprising European trade firms established offices and warehouses along the town's waterways during this time. Notable among these was the British-owned Heald Trading Company which commenced local operations in the 1860s. Its success later convinced a consortium of British industrialists that Dagupan could potentially become the most important trade post north of Manila. In 1887, they formed the *Ferrocaril de Manila-a-Dagupan* which secured the rights from the Spanish colonial government to develop the only direct railway between Manila and Central Luzon's northern coast (Basa 1997). Construction on the Manila-Dagupan Railroad commenced a year later and was finally completed in 1892. The steam locomotive's success helped solidify Dagupan's position as the region's dominant transport and trade center. Over succeeding decades, Dagupan enjoyed primacy as a major station for the flow of goods and people between the northern Philippines and Manila. This position was further solidified by the launch of the American-owned Pangasinan Transportation Company (Pantranco), a passenger bus line that facilitated travel throughout Pangasinan and beyond (Vistro and Reyes 2005:96–97).

The first three decades of the twentieth century—following the Philippine Revolution (1896–1898) and establishment of the U.S. colonial government during the American-Filipino Conflict (1898–1902)—Dagupan's socioeconomic and commercial landscape became more complex. Population increases and infrastructure improvements to the local built environment and road, bridge, and rail networks further integrated the town into the regional, national, and global economy. By 1938, Dagupan not only boasted some 36,000 inhabitants but its downtown began assuming a much more urban character. Low-rise wooden buildings were gradually replaced by multistory concrete commercial structures.

The traumas and setbacks fostered by three years of Japanese occupation during World War II were somewhat ameliorated following the ratification of Dagupan's cityhood charter in 1947 (Vistro and Reyes 2005:115). During the post-war decades stretching roughly from 1950 to 1990, the city underwent continued demographic and socioeconomic expansion. The local population nearly tripled from approximately 44,000 in 1948 to upwards of 122,000 in 1990 (Basa 1997). The launch of various hospitals, colleges and universities, public marketplaces, hotels, car dealerships, lumberyards, small groceries, and department stores occurred alongside these years of population growth.

Today, Dagupan boasts a vibrant, if sometimes hectic, downtown that stands in contrast with the more subdued and rural character of its outlying districts and neighborhoods. The city proper sits along a stretch of low-lying land intersected by seven rivers and 14 creeks that variously converge and empty into the Lingayen Gulf. The *población* is bisected by two main commercial roadways—A. B. Fernandez Avenue and Perez Boulevard—that are prone to flooding during the rainy season and lined with various mid- to low-rise buildings with traditional street store operations on the first floor and living accommodations and storage facilities above. Although not as rampant as in years past, local pedestrians continue to compete for sidewalk space with scores of food and dry-goods vendors who ply their wares to passers-by during normal business hours.

Moving away from this bustling sphere of activity and commerce, the pace and intensity of local life markedly slackens. Indeed, Dagupan's less urbanized *barangays* (municipal districts akin to neighborhoods) exhibit a number of distinctive features that stand in contrast to what is typically encountered in the *población*. The public infrastructure found in these outlying districts is noticeably less developed relative to downtown. While urban Dagupan encompasses a central business district that includes a network of east-west business thoroughfares and secondary streets frequently congested with pedestrian and vehicular traffic, its rural periphery features more of a patchwork of manmade fishponds and rice paddies that define the built morphology of those agricultural areas to the east, west, and south of the downtown business core. The local aquaculture industry is dedicated primarily to the raising of those small silver-scaled milkfish known as bangus. So well-known is this sector of Dagupan's traditional economy, in fact, that the city holds a local bangus festival each year to celebrate this adopted symbol of municipal identity.

Like other towns and cities in the Philippines, local commerce in Dagupan generally corresponds to the dichotomous formal/informal economic model whereby a limited but growing number of highly capitalized formal enterprises operate alongside scores of micro and small-scale informal ventures within the several public marketplace buildings. Dagupan's formal sector of urban retailing is effectively dominated by a small but influential community of Chinese-Filipinos whose local roots date back to the nineteenth century. While comprising less than 5 percent of Dagupeños, this close-knit group has remained at the forefront of downtown's street store trade for generations—especially in sub-sectors like groceries, textiles, hardware, and appliances—and on average their firms are more highly capitalized than those of the ethnic Filipinos (Dannhaeuser 2004; Lim 1997).

In part, this business supremacy is facilitated by the coordinated efforts of the local Chinese Chamber of Commerce and the more recent participation of Chinese-Filipino business owners in city and provincial government. Indeed, the last two city mayors have been Chinese-Filipinos with considerable business pedigrees in the local grocery and shopping mall trade. In fact, two of the largest malls in greater Dagupan are owned and operated respectively by these commercial and political opponents. Perhaps more so than anyone else, these two individuals and their respective retail firms are most responsible for revolutionizing the ways locals purchase and consume food. Indeed, through their official and business decisions both of these local politicians have wielded considerable influence over the character and direction of local retailing in the 1990s, 2000s, and beyond. Their municipal policies and commercial rivalries have helped blunt the reach of some large Manila-based shopping mall developers looking to establish a presence in greater Dagupan over the years just as they have expedited franchising opportunities in and around downtown that largely benefited their political and economic interests.

Against this backdrop, it is probably unsurprising that most of the firms engaged in Dagupan's burgeoning fast food scene came from the local Chinese-Filipino trade community (Dannhaeuser 2004). Thanks to the efforts and significant capital resources of a few enterprising ethnic Chinese family firms, national and international fast food brands headquartered in Metro-Manila were able to either gain a significant foothold or solidify their position in local commerce. So, even as most everyday restaurant staff are comprised of college-age Filipinos, the operators of McDonald's, Jollibee, and, indeed, all of the major players in Dagupan's fast food scene come from this small but economically and politically vital minority community.

While securing the rights to manage such global and homegrown chains at the community level often leads to sizable profits, it does not necessarily translate into full control over daily operations. To be sure, the overarching Manila-based master franchise holders do much to set the tone and parameters of how their provincial enterprises operate. This control effectively limits the role of local fast food franchisees in Dagupan and elsewhere in terms of innovation and creativity. Franchisees mainly serve in a supervisory capacity. They rarely deviate from guiding company principles on how to produce, serve, and market fast food to local diners. For example, franchise hiring practices basically conform to those policies coming out of Manila whereby most wage-earners are only employed for a five-month contract so as to avoid providing the health and other job benefits available to long-term employees (Dannhaeuser 2004:142).

The specifics of the relationship between those Manila-based firms holding fast food master franchises and their local affiliates notwithstanding, the rise of national and international chain eateries in provincial Philippine communities like Dagupan can be seen as benefiting from other retail developments. Indeed, the penetration of American-style quick-service eateries unfolded in parallel with the emergence of several modern department stores, supermarkets, malls, and warehouse clubs that were primarily located within the city center before radiating outward to the urban periphery. The success of these retail operations obviously could not have occurred without the market demand of an increasingly savvy consumer population now steeped in matters of fast food and mass consumption.

## DAGUPAN'S FAST FOOD SCENE (1980s–2010s)

Corporate fast food first appeared in Dagupan during the early 1980s with the launch of a few small multinational eateries, most notably Dunkin' Donuts and Shakey's Pizza, in or around the city center. The initial Shakey's went out of business in less than a year only to remerge later under new management in a different downtown location (Dannhaeuser 2004:140). Over subsequent years, several other national and transnational chains opened franchise or branch outlets in the *población*, including Dagupan's original Jollibee restaurant, which was strategically located along the city's main business thoroughfare A. B. Fernandez Avenue. This two-story eatery proved an almost immediate hit with local diners. Its success did much to convince other business firms that teaming up with well-known fast food brands was a financially sound undertaking.

Throughout the mid-to-late 1980s, fast food expansion occurred at a steady but not necessarily accelerated pace. During this period, the local dining scene continued to be dominated by a few sit-down restaurants that were usually affiliated with a downtown hotel and served traditional Filipino or Chinese fare. Such establishments featured table service and offered cuisine generally priced beyond the affordability of most everyday Dagupeños. Chief among these eateries was Dagupeña, a well-known local restaurant located within a historical building along A. B. Fernandez Avenue from the late 1920s until the early 2000s (Vistro and Reyes 2005:100). Among other things, Dagupeña housed two dining areas; one climate-controlled and the other without air-conditioning. Both were adorned with striking black and white photographs that traced Dagupan's historical development over the years.

Some of the multinational chains that appeared during the 1980s were Mister Donut and Cindy's Restaurant, the latter of which was basically a Filipino take on the classic American diner concept, with a menu featuring hot dogs, hamburgers, and French fries alongside some traditional indigenous dishes. In part, the limited availability of viable commercial space in the city center, coupled with a consumer population still somewhat lacking in purchasing power, constrained this initial period of chain restaurant growth. Since most retail activity remained concentrated downtown during this time, the prospects of new businesses opening outside the *población* were not widely embraced as economically viable.

One of the few exceptions to this trend was the mobile hamburger stands established by small fast food companies likes L. C. Big Mak, Frank'N Burger, and Burger Machine (Dannhaeuser 2004:234–235). These homegrown chains established several outdoor eateries in greater Dagupan near bus terminals, outlying *barangays*, or along stretches of highway leading out of town. Operationally, such modest 24/7 restaurants function somewhere between a traditional *carinderia* and a food truck. With no-frills menus, basic kitchen equipment and refrigeration, and simple counter seating of six to twelve stools, they mainly serve a clientele of pedestrians, night owls, students, or bus passengers. If the Philippines corporate fast food scene has a bottom tier for franchising opportunities, it is surely comprised of those outdoor burger stands operated by the likes of L. C. Big Mak, Frank'N Burger, and Burger Machine. With lower franchising fees, somewhere around ₱250,000 ($5,200) native Filipinos are more actively engaged relative to Chinese-Filipinos in this part of the fast food market sector.

The limited penetration of mobile burger stands in the urban periphery notwithstanding, sentiments about the economic viability of downtown persisted throughout the late 1980s. Such notions changed following a major earthquake in July 1990 when much of the urban core was destroyed or deemed uninhabitable. Although this disaster devastated local commerce in greater Dagupan over the short term, it also created a vacuum that brought about wholesale changes to the urban fabric. That is, it quickly ushered in a period of sustained retail modernization whereby older and more run-down structures were replaced with newer and more consumer-friendly ventures. Of note, it was during this period of recovery that various modern supermarket facilities opened their doors to local consumers.

In terms of scale and conspicuity, the opening of three large-scale shopping malls in greater Dagupan during this post-disaster period were perhaps most notable. While two of these enterprises were launched under the auspices of the family firm of Dagupan's current mayor, the other was established by her predecessor in municipal office. Not only did these competing consumer facilities significantly alter the character of the city's economic landscape, they also housed popular eateries such as Goldilocks, Chowking, Greenwich Pizza, McDonald's, KFC, Kenny Rogers' Roasters, Red Ribbon, and Jollibee. Unlike the dining options available at most enclosed shopping centers in the United States or even Metro-Manila, the quick-service eateries located within Dagupan's various mall enterprises are not organized collectively around a centralized food court where customers order food at one of several restaurant service counters and then take their trays to a table or booth within a communal area for sit-down dining. Rather, these fast food operations generally occupy first floor locations at or near the mall foyer and feature glassed walls that look out on both the outside and mall interiors.

Even with these prime spots located in such close proximity to these high-traffic pedestrian areas, most mall eateries also include access doors of their own leading to the outside. These smaller entrances are typically maintained by uniformed security guards who, besides projecting an air of visible authority, also greet or assist customers as well as log employees in and out when work shifts change. Oftentimes, these armed personnel stand behind a speaker's podium where they keep an eye on comings and goings both within and outside the restaurant. Whether male or female, the multiplicity of gun-toting guards encountered at quick-service eateries, shopping malls, and other retail establishments throughout the Philippines serves ostensibly as a proactive deterrent to would-be lawbreakers but in actuality approaches something akin to "security theater," whereby such conspicuous countermeasure heighten feelings of perceived crime and instability without doing much toward actually improving public safety (Schneier 2003:38).

Generally speaking, Dagupan's mall fast food outlets are smaller than their stand-alone counterparts both in terms of kitchen space and seating capacity. In this way, they tend to feature fewer consumer amenities like party rooms, playgrounds, and karaoke systems. In some cases, plastic picnic tables and chairs are set up within the mall itself. Such seating just outside of the restaurant is useful to accommodate customer overflows during peak business hours.

By 2005, there were some 40 fast food eateries—representing 13 distinct national and transnational brands—operating in and around downtown Dagupan. Among these were four Jollibee restaurants, two Chowkings, and three McDonald's, all located within short traveling distance of the city's three major universities: the University of Pangasinan, the University of Luzon, and the Colegio de Dagupan. Perhaps as anticipated, these establishments quickly emerged as popular hangouts for students during much of the school week as they offered opportunities for socializing and dining occurred in almost equal measure. Indeed, rare is the weekday afternoon when these eateries are not teeming with packs of undergraduate Dagupeños crowded around restaurant seating over soft drinks and assorted menu items.

With such growth in corporate fast food, it is important to recognize other local dining options that remain available both within and beyond Dagupan proper. Street food, traditional sit-down restaurants, and take-out from *carinderias* or canteens, among other possibilities, still serve as viable alternatives for those looking to eat outside the home. That said, the appearance of McDonald's, Jollibee, and other quick-services eateries alongside other changes in the urban fabric has undeniably affected the ways locals eat.

While never directly competing with the city's emerging fast food scene, the aforementioned Dagupeña and other longtime restaurants either went out of business or relocated away from the *población* as the character of urban life assumed a more sterilized or corporatized edge. With fewer non-chain eateries in and around Dagupan's city center from which to choose, local diners must now invest more time, effort, and travel to enjoy authentic sit-down cuisine. In the case of Dagupeña, the restaurant moved to a new site several kilometers away from downtown in the nearby community of Calasiao. Notably, the historical building it occupied for decades was razed to make way for a modern-looking commercial complex that sits rather incongruously among neighboring shops and businesses given its height and uniquely postmodern design. With each passing year, its steel and glass façade looks more and more weathered and out of place amid its immediate surroundings.

Since 2005, the number of quick-service eateries in greater Dagupan has effectively doubled although some established brands had subsequently moved to new commercial sites. For example, Jollibee's flagship store operating at the east end of A. B. Fernandez Avenue switched corner locations around this busy downtown intersection at least three times since the mid-1990s. In fact, it seemed that on every trip that I made to Dagupan from the late 1990s onward, this particular Jollibee would have moved from one part of the intersection to the opposite side. As if following suit, the second McDonald's outlet to open in Dagupan occupied a commercial space near this same high-traffic junction for a few years before moving a block or so north to a lot fronting the University of Pangasinan.

## FAST FOOD FAILURES—DAGUPAN CITY (2000s)

Despite the overall growth and popularity of corporate fast food in Dagupan since the 1980s not all brands have achieved sufficient staying power within this increasingly cutthroat restaurant scene. While most well-known national and international chains have succeeded in satisfying the tastes and sensibilities of local consumers, there have been a few quick-service eateries that launched franchise or branch outlets to much fanfare and press coverage only to shutter operations within less than a year. This inability to cultivate or sustain a loyal customer base is perhaps best exemplified the demise of two different Manila-based restaurant companies in the mid-2000s: the more popular American brand A&W Restaurant and the less familiar homegrown chain Hen Lin, a Chinese quick-service eatery specializing in *dim sum* (steamed or fried dumplings served with various fillings as snacks or meals). In both cases, a range of internal and external factors lead to their respective closings.

In December 2003 a gleaming new A&W Restaurant opened for business along a heavily traveled stretch of Perez Boulevard near the approach slab of a multilane bridge spanning the Pantal River. The launch of this soft drink–inspired eatery commenced with a ribbon-cutting ceremony attended by the local Chinese-Filipino franchise holder as well as a company representative from the United States. Besides a stationary menu comprised of American fast food favorites including hamburgers and French fries, not to mention more surprising offerings such as pizza and spaghetti, the two-story restaurant also boasted an ample parking lot and automobile drive-thru lane. In an apparent bid to attract the increasing number of Dagupeños who now owned private vehicles, these sorts of consumer amenities represented a first for downtown Dagupan's established restaurant scene. Indeed, since the A&W seemed to promise a new phase in the development of local fast food retailing, its closing some six months later was not something readily anticipated.

The restaurant's lack of appeal among city diners can be attributed to various factors. For one thing, many locals simply did not appreciate the ingredients and flavors associated with A&W's standard bill of fare. The overall impression that the restaurant's menu instilled was one whereby the familiar sweet and succulent tastes that Filipinos generally favor were subordinated to those decidedly more sharp and tangy flavors that traditionally resonate with American palates. Even though the chain had successfully established outlets in other parts of the country, the A&W brand failed to connect with local appetites in any meaningful way.

After the restaurant's initial novelty wore off, few diners were so fond of A&W so as to be considered repeat customers. Beyond simple matters of taste, A&W products were also slightly more expensive than comparable menu items sold by the likes of McDonald's and Jollibee. All things considered, customers generally liked A&W's root beer, ice cream floats, and other desserts but not much else. This limited appeal did not translate into high profit margins. Thus, in a local fast food scene where established chains offered more familiar tastes and lower prices, the margin for error for a lesser known restaurant brand like A&W was rather limited.

A&W's inability to gain a sufficient foothold among motorists and other key segments of Dagupan's dining public was a blow from which the enterprise was never able to recover. As noted above, the eatery operated through a franchise agreement between the A&W Company headquartered in Metro-Manila and a Chinese-Filipino franchise holder whose rental arrangement with a local property owner necessitated a steady stream of income to meet regular overhead costs. With his dwindling consumer base and declining profits, he could not keep up with the high monthly rental fees that approached ₱100,000 (approximately $2,100). By summer 2004, the underperforming restaurant quietly went out of business. The once sleek and sophisticated fast food eatery remained shuttered for the next several years before finally reemerging as the site of a new 7-Eleven convenience store.

Following in the wake of the A&W Restaurant's untimely demise in downtown Dagupan is the equally brief existence of a Hen Lin location several blocks away. As another, albeit less conspicuous, example of a nationally known chain eatery failing to survive the city's expanding fast food scene in the mid-2000s, this Hong Kong-style *dim sum* eatery commenced operations along the city's main business thoroughfare of A. B. Fernandez Avenue in 2004. Besides its specialized bill of fare, Hen Lin also offered selections of *siapao* (noodles), spaghetti, and fried chicken. At first glance, the enterprise seemed poised for success given its ideal location along the city's busiest pedestrian strip and proximity to so many street stores with Chinese-Filipino owner-operators.

Hen Lin traces its roots back to the early 1980s when a small mom-and-pop Chinese eatery located in the Paranaque district of Metro-Manila started selling its affordable cuisine to fast food patrons. Over the years, Hen Lin expanded operations with mall food kiosks and stand-alone eateries throughout Luzon. The company logo of a pudgy smiling Chinese chef had become a familiar sight to thousands of everyday Filipinos. So, despite indications suggesting that its operations in Dagupan would approach a level of success comparable to Hen Lin branches and franchises elsewhere, such outcomes never really materialized. Indeed, by summer 2005, the inaugural Hen Lin store had ceased operations. In part, this failure was precipitated by the restaurant's very limited seating capacity and distinct lack of ambience. Compared to the amenities available at the neighboring Jollibee, KFC, and McDonald's, Hen Lin was just not in the same league.

Speaking from personal experience I remember passing by the eatery one summer morning in 2005, noticing a few diners milling about with nothing out of the ordinary going on. The very next day the entire store was being gutted by a crew of workers with bandanas wrapped around their faces. Amid considerable noise and dust, restaurant fixtures, signage, seating, and other accoutrements were stripped out of the commercial space to make way for a new retail venture. Within a matter of days, an entirely different business dealing in women's ready-to-wear clothing occupied the site. To passers-by unfamiliar with the location's previous tenet, it was as if the Manila-based *dim sum* eatery never existed.

In retrospect, the particularly short-lived cases of Dagupan's A&W and Hen Lin suggest that the popularity of corporate fast food in the provincial Philippines faces certain limits that cannot be overcome simply through novelty and flashy aesthetics. Without the considerable brand appeal of more established chains, smaller quick-service eateries can sometimes overextend themselves in ways that prove unsustainable for the long term. This is especially true as the number of corporate fast food outlets and brands continues to expand.

## FAST FOOD INNOVATIONS—DAGUPAN CITY (2000s–2010s)

The lack of staying power exhibited by A&W, Hen Lin, and a few other quick-service eateries including Dagupan's only Kenny Rogers' Roasters (a mall location) was more than offset by various expansions and innovations in other areas of the city's fast food scene. In some cases, such developments took the form of new consumer amenities that helped expand local dining options or facilitate customer transactions. In other instances, they involved structural renovations to existing restaurants or the introduction of new chains with decidedly different approaches to how consumers utilize their retail space.

In the early 2000s, all McDonald's and Jollibee locations in Dagupan gave diners the option to purchase food orders using credit cards. Scanners were installed near cash registers along the service counter where cardholders could easily swipe their plastic currency. While this convenient form of payment helped expedite over-the-counter transactions, it really only affected a narrow subset of customers since most everyday Filipinos lacked credit cards. Besides this new method of payment, both chains also began offering free delivery to those customers and households who phoned, texted, or placed their orders in person with the restaurants beforehand. Once this service went into effect, the sight of mopeds and scooters crowded along restaurant parking lots became almost as common as that of jumpsuited fast food employees zipping through local traffic.

Having utilized this service on occasion, I can offer some insights into the finer points of having fast food delivered in this manner. In July 2005, a week or so before my scheduled return to the United States, my friend and research assistant Mario and I decided to throw a small get-together for family and acquaintances as a gesture of thanks. Mario lived on the outskirts of Dagupan not far from the beach but still some kilometers away from the nearest fast food restaurant. Thus, we opted to have some Jollibee delivered to his residence. Since we were feeding upwards of 15 people, we decided to keep things simple by ordering pretty much the same thing for everyone. For what initially appeared as a rather straightforward undertaking, an unusual series of steps and interactions with restaurant staff were required to effectively see this transaction through. Maybe if we had only placed an order for one or two diners, this task would not have become so unnecessarily complicated.

At the time of our event, Jollibee did not make delivery menus available to customers. Similarly, Internet service and smart phones were not widely available for online orders. Thus, Mario and I went to Jollibee's flagship store on east A. B. Fernandez Avenue a few days before the party to arrange the delivery of eight Yum! Meals and eight Kiddie Meals, comprised of potato chips, hamburgers, soft drinks and, in the case of the latter, small plastic toys. Unbeknownst to us, take-out deliveries's bags of potato chips are substituted for French fries to ensure freshness and prevent spillage. Mario's protests that we were entitled to a discount because of this practice pretty much went nowhere with the store manager. We made arrangements for them to call us before the party at 2:30 pm to confirm our delivery. We even provided them a hand-drawn map to avoid any unnecessary confusion.

At ten minutes to two on the day of the party, Mario received a phone call from the Jollibee manager asking if we did indeed want to go through with the order. He confirmed, and nearly 15 minutes later the driver wheeled his moped into a makeshift driveway not far from an adjacent printing press. At this point, he began unpacking the contents of a durable plastic cooler attached directly behind the scooter's seat. All of the same items were packed together in plastic Jollibee bags so that hamburgers, chips, and soft drinks were kept separate. Drinks came in plastic cups with the lids taped down while straws, ketchup, and napkins were individually sorted. Significantly, the Yum! Burgers were still warm to the touch thanks to their transport in an insulated container. Upon paying the driver, several neighbors showed up to congratulate me, thinking it was my birthday. For this outlying neighborhood, apparently one of the few if only times fast food is ordered in this quantity or delivery method is for the occasion of a birthday celebration.

Beyond free delivery, a few other innovations were introduced exclusively by McDonald's in and around Dagupan. While the Golden Arches still trailed Jollibee in terms of popularity (Matejowsky 2009), the chain did variously tweak its local operations to entice customers in somewhat novel ways. For example, the company launched a small dessert kiosk in the mid-2000s

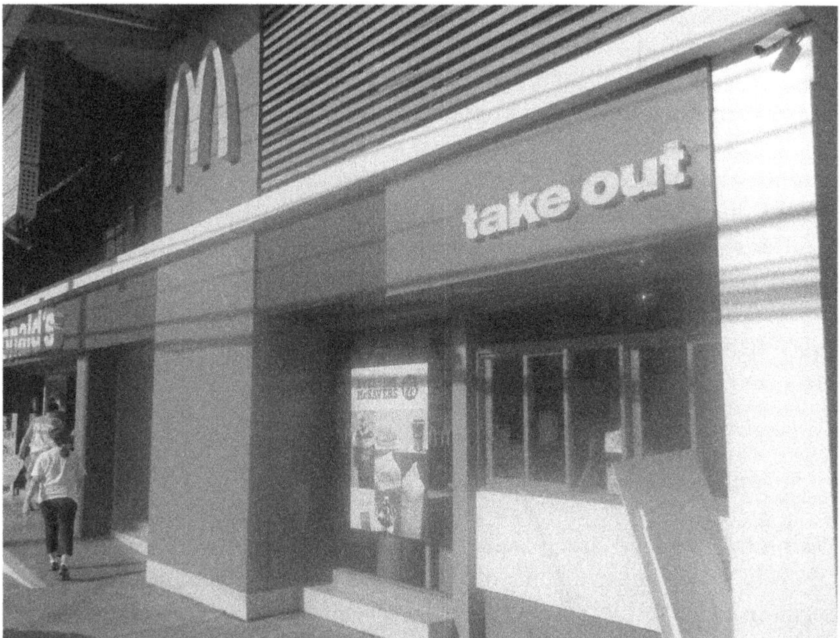


**Figure 3.1 McDonald's with Take Out Window, Dagupan City 2015.** Photo taken by Ty Matejowsky.

near the entrance of a warehouse club and giant shopping mall west of the *población* and owned by the current mayor. In a way, this modest restaurant stall acts as an extension of the busy McDonald's eatery situated on the other side of the two-story shopping center. The air-conditioned kiosk is hard to miss given its colorful paint job and location underneath the mall's covered drop-off zone. Jeepney and tricycle (hired motorcycles with sidecars) passengers seem to like it as they can load up on ice cream and other frozen desserts before or after their daily commute.

Seemingly building off this innovation, the new McDonald's located just outside the main gate of the University of Pangasinan recently installed a convenient walk-up window that operates something like a drive-thru service for passers-by. This modified restaurant design allows pedestrians to place and receive take-out orders without ever stepping inside the eatery. The customer queue for this newfound offering usually gets pretty long right around *merienda* time when college students begin spilling out of class in search of a quick snack. At such times, the already congested sidewalks fronting the school become even more crowded. The throngs of undergraduate Dagupeños that utilize this service soon give way to those heading home in the early evening.

Beyond just snacks, these patrons are looking to grab hamburgers or other meals-on-the-go for their spouses and children. Even after this dinnertime rush dissipates, the walk-up window remains open for business. In fact, during late-night hours, it serves something of a dual purpose because it allows sales to continue while also providing a measure of security for restaurant employees. In this way it is somewhat similar to the transparent bulletproof partitions favored by convenience store operations in some high crime areas in the United States.

Offering continuous restaurant innovations and services like those mentioned above now stands as a key feature of Dagupan's fast food scene. Competing restaurant brands are always on the lookout for ways to distinguish themselves from rivals as well as appeal to a consumer base increasingly savvy about the latest retail trends and offerings.

## STARBUCKS RISING—DAGUPAN CITY (2010s)

With local fast food preferences still leaning heavily toward Jollibee given the chain's deep understanding of Filipino palates, it seemed that McDonald's began using other approaches at its disposal including dessert kiosks and walk-up windows to close the gap with its primary competitor. Adding new dimension to this ongoing burger rivalry was the more recent appearance of another popular global chain in downtown Dagupan. Indeed, possibly the most conspicuous and highly capitalized entry into the local fast food scene in the 2010s is the new Starbucks located along west A. B. Fernandez Avenue in a shopping plaza across the street from the recently refurbished municipal hall.

While not a quick-service eatery in the strictest sense, the Seattle-based coffeehouse does stand as one of the world's most recognizable consumer brands with its popular selection of gourmet warm/cold beverages, fresh/packaged food items, and java-inspired products. Although a few coffeehouse ventures have come and gone in Dagupan over the years—many of which were operated as cyber-cafés with rows and rows of noisy computer terminals dedicated primarily to online gaming—the new Starbucks boasted a much more quiet and relaxed atmosphere. It also featured various consumer amenities such as free Wi-Fi, piped music, and probably the cleanest bathrooms in greater Dagupan.

Starbucks has been in the Philippines since 1998, boasting over 200 locations nationwide. The coffeehouse that was launched locally in May 2014 was just the second company outlet to open its doors in Pangasinan. Significantly, the new venture operates not as a franchise but rather as a corporate branch. Though not openly competing with Jollibee, McDonald's and other top fast food sellers, per se, the java house brand does exert something of an indirect influence on the operations of various quick-service eateries at the local level.

This type of sway is surprising considering that Starbucks tends to attract customers with slightly more discretionary income than those frequenting the Philippines' top burger chains. Like their American counterparts, Filipino clientele tend to use Starbucks for more than just drinking coffee. Indeed, for many people the store serves as something of a hangout where friends can gather together over lattes or students or professionals can meet to casually work on projects. This is especially nice for the latter since the only other local venue for collaborative work is the Dagupan City Library which closes around 5 pm.

Both Jollibee and McDonald's ostensibly borrowed a page from Starbucks' corporate playbook in terms of aesthetics and ambience. Indeed, I was pleasantly surprised upon returning to Dagupan in 2015 to find both downtown McDonald's and to a lesser extent, the nearby Jollibee remodeled in ways that echoed the coffeehouse's stylish wood, glass, and chrome accents. On my last visit, the interiors of these Jollibee and McDonald's restaurants featured cheery paint schemes with bright primary colors, now these eateries sport an arguably more refined look with dark muted tones highlighted by sophisticated lighting and furnishings. While the likelihood of being confused with the understated décor of a chic five-star restaurant located in Manila is remote, the renovations of these quick-service eateries evoke a little more in terms of aesthetic refinement.

Moreover, the dining areas of Jollibee and McDonald's—which previously featured symmetrical rows of tables and booths set up to accommodate as many customers as possible—are currently arranged with much less uniformity. Dine-in customers now have more seating options available to them including low-slung padded stools, fixed dining counters, and movable table and chairs that can be combined or separated depending on party size. This flexible layout suggests more openness about how consumers utilize restaurant space, particularly those fast food patrons who are slow to leave once orders are consumed. This sort of tolerance reflects a departure from previous restaurant practices where staff applied a discernible pressure on diners to eat quickly and vacate seating so as to make way for others. Today, Dagupan's two main fast food eateries increasingly resemble Starbucks not just in appearance but in how they extend much more latitude to customers when it comes to lingering or hanging out.

Unlike peak coffee time in the United States, business hours at the new Starbucks in Dagupan remain rather slack for the first part of the day. Indeed, the place is noticeably quiet with more than half of the seats empty. Customers that do frequent the coffeehouse in the morning typically purchase some variety of hot or cold beverage served in the company's familiar disposable cups. After receiving their drinks, they usually depart without much in the way of hanging around. Notwithstanding the stray Australian tourist or Filipino retiree idling away some time, this pattern tends to repeat itself throughout most of the midday and afternoon.

Only toward the end of the workday as office personnel, students, and others finish up their duties and head over to the coffeehouse does business start to pick up. By the time evening rolls around, the Starbucks is humming with activity. So popular is the coffeehouse during these times that it is not uncommon to experience an almost standing-room-only vibe in the place. With free Internet service, the coffeehouse attracts scores of young professionals and college types who remain glued to their smartphones as they crowd around the raised tables and cushioned couches and chairs. The counter crew sporting green aprons and hats keep busy filling orders and busing tables. All in all, it is difficult to find a livelier nightspot outside of the bars and discos dotting the roads leading out to Dagupan's coastal *barangays*.

In this regard, Starbucks offers trend-conscious Dagupeños a viable alternative to the fast food offerings of McDonald's, Jollibee, and other top brands. Unsurprisingly, its success has spurred these established quick-service eateries to alter or reformulate some aspects of their operations. Whether or not Starbucks continues to exert this sort of influence over Dagupan's fast food scene in the near or distant future remains to be seen. That said, growth in this sector of the city's retail economy shows no real signs of slowing down. The way things now stand, it is hard to imagine Dagupan City without its various fast food restaurants.

## SAN FERNANDO CITY, LA UNION—HISTORY AND SOCIOECONOMIC STRUCTURE

San Fernando is a coastal city of over 120,000 inhabitants located nearly 280 kilometers north of Metro-Manila and some 85 kilometers north of Dagupan City. The city occupies a west-central section of the province of La Union along the area where the Lingayen Gulf merges into the South China Sea. Its physical topography is characterized by coastal lowlands and a mountainous interior.

Before it fell under Spanish rule in the later sixteenth century, San Fernando's current site was occupied by three indigenous settlements (History of San Fernando 1983:23). Internecine tribal warfare and occasional pirate raids characterized much of native life during pre-Hispanic times. After gaining a sufficient foothold in the area during the early seventeenth century, Spanish colonial administrators condensed these three villages into one centralized location to better protect against external threats. Despite two uprisings in 1660 and 1762, colonial officials established a rather extended period of peace and order that lasted well into the nineteenth century.

During this time, early San Fernando emerged as one of the provincial Philippines' chief outposts for tobacco cultivation (Meimban 1997). This cash crop's export did much to integrate what until this time was a relatively isolated community into the regional and national economy. Also crucial to San Fernando's ongoing ascension was its declaration as the capital of the newly created La Union province in 1850. With a population of some 4,800 inhabitants in 1850, daily life in San Fernando remained somewhat more austere relative to what was encountered in neighboring Dagupan, Pangasinan. From the mid-1800s onwards, San Fernando underwent various infrastructural improvements. Besides expansion of the town's existing road and bridge network, a rudimentary highway system leading into the eastern rugged interior was completed. This development, coupled with pier renovation along the community's natural harbor, did much to enhance the town's role in regional and maritime trade (Meimban 1997).

Around the twentieth century's outset, San Fernando's political economy experienced profound changes resulting from events rooted in the Philippine Revolution (1896–1898) and American-Filipino Conflict (1898–1902). A brief period of self-rule following the overthrow of La Union's Spanish magistrate in 1898 was cut short with the arrival of U.S. troops to the region in 1899. The American military soon defeated local freedom fighters and converted the area in and around San Fernando into a garrison town. Consistent with happenings in other parts of the Philippines, the four decades preceding World War II marked a critical period in San Fernando's urban and socioeconomic development. Numerous elementary and secondary schools, hospitals, government buildings, banking institutions were constructed at the local level alongside the town's first movie theater and family-style restaurant. Moreover a Catholic college was launched in 1910 and in 1929 the town became the northern terminal of an extension of the Manila-Dagupan railway. Electrification of downtown and the installation of a rudimentary sewer system followed in the 1930s (Meimban 1997:205–208).

The Japanese invasion and subsequent repatriation of the Philippines during World War II caused considerable damage to the town's existing infrastructure. Post-war years witnessed an accelerated period of rebuilding and urbanization. Coinciding with such improvements was increased demographic growth. San Fernando's population rose nearly threefold from approximately 29,000 to nearly 85,000 in 1990. By the early 1980s, the municipal trade sector had effectively come into its own as an important center of regional commerce. The total number of registered businesses operating in and around San Fernando's *población* had increased substantially since the 1950s. Numerous multinational corporations including Coca-Cola, Pepsi-Cola, and Philip Morris had established warehouse and distribution centers in the greater San Fernando area just as several department stores and modest supermarkets emerged locally. In many ways, these developments seemed to anticipate the arrival of corporate fast food restaurants in the mid-1990s.

Today, most San Fernandians live in one of the 20 low-lying *barangays* paralleling the north-south shoreline. Given its seaside locale and white sandy beaches, San Fernando serves as a well-known tourist destination for foreign and domestic travelers. Especially popular is the string of holiday resorts just south of the city. Of almost equal appeal—particularly to the international surfing set—are the various coastal spots a few kilometers north of the city near the town of San Juan.

As a bustling but orderly tertiary city, downtown San Fernando is geographically situated between a deep water harbor that reflects the city's historical maritime orientation and the abruptly rocky terrain of the Cordillera mountain chain. Like other towns and cities in the Philippines, the layout of downtown San Fernando adheres to a grid system whereby a series of east-west and north-south streets and thoroughfares encompass a municipal core comprised of the three major features of traditional urban Hispanicization: the town plaza, city hall, and local Catholic Church complex. Surrounding this urban core is a mismatch of modern and older mid- to low-rise buildings that comprises the *población*'s street-level fabric.

Overlooking all of this are La Union's Provincial Capitol building and ornate Chinese Friendship Pagoda. From the vantage point of these elevated structures high atop a jagged mountain peak, it is easy to trace the route of a well-traveled road known as the National Highway that bisects the city center and is lined with various signage for fast food companies including

McDonald's, KFC, Jollibee, and Pizza Hut. This sometimes congested transportation artery connects the less densely populated and remote areas of the northern Philippines to the more urbanized territories of Central and Southern Luzon. As it cuts through downtown, this stretch of road is dubbed Quezon Avenue.

No less visible from this lofty lookout is the tongue of land that juts out into the South China Sea several kilometers before curving backwards on itself to create the harbor's southern rim. Known as Poro Point, the peninsula's extreme tip was long home to a small U.S. military base first called Camp Wallace in 1903 and then subsequently changed to the Wallace Air Station. For the past quarter-century, the site has functioned as a center of operations for the Philippine Navy. Among various docking facilities, Poro Point also features a sizable radar installation as well as a nine-hole golf course that has fallen into disrepair.

Given its geographic location and accessibility, San Fernando serves as the primary trade, governmental, financial, health care, and educational hub for the province of La Union. More broadly, it also operates as the administrative seat for Region One, a multi-provincial development zone comprised of Pangasinan, La Union, Ilocos Sur, and Ilocos Norte. Within this official capacity, downtown San Fernando is comprised of blocks of various mid-rise buildings that house almost as many retail shops and businesses as they do municipal, provincial, and regional government offices. Since many office workers live outside of the city, San Fernando's downtown population tends to fluctuate significantly depending on whether or not it is a weekday. Accordingly, commercial business tends to spike during the workweek and recede somewhat on Saturdays and Sundays.

Most of those living in and around San Fernando proper claim an Ilocano heritage. Ilocanos represent the third largest ethnic group in the Philippines and are traditionally recognized for their hard-working, frugal, and enterprising tendencies (Pertierra 1995). So much so, in fact, that they are often linked with other stereotypically parsimonious groups like the Scots (Pertierra 1995). Like neighboring Dagupan City, San Fernando is also home to a small but powerful non-indigenous group that has figured prominently in local affairs since the mid-nineteenth century. San Fernando's ethnic Chinese community has contributed to the city's rise in numerous ways. Nowhere is this more evident than in matters of municipal trade. This tight-knit community has remained at the forefront of area commerce for generations even though they have never made up more than 5 percent of the total population. Broadly speaking, most highly capitalized commercial enterprises in San Fernando have owner-operators with Chinese ancestry. With few exceptions, this sort of ethnic affiliation tends to find representation in the city's increasingly prosperous fast food scene.

## SAN FERNANDO'S FAST FOOD SCENE (1980s–2010s)

By the late 1980s, several modern supermarkets, department stores, and appliance/electronics showrooms were operating in San Fernando's *población.* Most occupied shopfronts along Quezon Avenue or in those street store spaces that looked onto the central public marketplace at the heart of downtown. For the most part, these establishments catered to a clientele comprised of middle-class professionals and households with some level of economic affluence. It was also around this time that corporate fast food first appeared on the local scene, albeit, in a rather muted way. Multinational fast food brands Dunkin' Donuts and Mister Donut opened outlets in the city center as did homegrown American-style diner chain Cindy's.

In terms of floor space and consumer amenities, these eateries did not have much to offer. Limited seating and a no-frills ambience contributed to local perceptions that these ventures were basically novelties with little prospect of long-term future success. Accordingly, Cindy's went out of business after only a few years of operation due to insufficient patronage. So, rather than ushering in a new period of fast food expansion, the arrival of Dunkin' Donuts, Mister Donut, and Cindy's merely hinted at what would later become an enhanced trend of chain restaurant growth. Indeed, several years would pass before this type of fare would catch on and fast food companies could begin expanding their San Fernando operations. For the time being, the local dining scene remained defined by the various Chinese restaurants operating downtown as well as several sit-down establishments associated with the nearby holiday resorts.

San Fernando experienced a major surge of retail expansion in the mid-1990s. The opening of a bi-level strip mall along the National Highway just south of the *población* in early 1996 marked a turning point for urban commercial growth. Dubbed the Christ the King College (CKC) Commercial Center, the retail complex was owned by the local Catholic diocese under the auspices of its private college whose campus was located directly across the highway. Among other things, the shopping center quickly became a focal point for the next stage of fast food expansion at the community level.

A Mister Donut eatery occupied a store space at the strip mall's southern edge while a Giacomino's Pizza and Pasta was housed at the shopping plaza's opposite end. The new Mister Donut outlet was virtually identical to the firm's downtown branch in that it was rather small with few consumer amenities, while the more spacious Giacomino's operated as a modern pizzeria similar in style to the homegrown chain Greenwich Pizza or global leader Pizza Hut. For all the possibilities and novelty of these strip mall eateries, their locations just beyond the reach of downtown limited their consumer appeal somewhat. It would only be a matter of months, however, until the full impact of corporate fast food would be felt at the local level.

Indeed, 1997 marked a crucial turning point for San Fernando's burgeoning fast food scene. Three of the nation's largest fast food brands—McDonald's, Jollibee, and Chowking—set up operations in or around the urban core following the CKC Commercial Center's successful launch. Over the course of several months in spring 1997, the city's commercial landscape came to include these popular eateries with locations along or near the National Highway (Quezon Avenue). Of little surprise, the restaurants were quite similar with regard to service style, consumer amenities, sanitary conditions, and indoor layouts. Variations were present, however, in terms of size, exterior design, menu selection, and primary clientele. The emergence of corporate fast food in San Fernando—such differences and similarities notwithstanding—altered the local urban fabric in ways still being felt today.

## McDONALD'S—SAN FERNANDO CITY (1990s–2010s)

The first major chain to open its doors locally was McDonald's. In June 1997, the Golden Arches launched a new restaurant just opposite the CKC Commercial Center several blocks south of downtown. The venture represented McDonald's initial incursion into La Union though most locals were already familiar with the brand as the company had been in the Philippines since 1981. For bus and jeepney travelers heading northbound along the National Highway, one of the first sights to catch their attention upon approaching San Fernando is the company's iconic red and gold logo. It towers meters-high above nearby businesses and rooflines. In this way, it serves as a vivid reminder of how a lack of enforceable zoning laws at the community level informs the character of urban centers across the provincial Philippines.

The events leading up to McDonald's first appearance in San Fernando readily align with the company's strategy of partnering with local firms and individuals as much as possible (Watson 1997:12). Again, this approach entails the U.S.-based McDonald's—through its overseas master franchise holder McGeorge Food Industries—contracting with a local individual or firm to run the restaurant for a period of no less than ten years. Under this arrangement, the prospective partner puts up a substantial franchise fee and locates a property capable of housing the restaurant facility. In some instances, a market feasibility study conducted by the franchisee is required before contract negotiations can move forward.

Once the franchise agreement is finalized, the local operator takes charge of the restaurant's daily operations and pays the company an adjustable monthly rental. With at least a 40–50 percent stake in its international operations, the

McDonald's Corporation is able to exact compliance from its franchise holders with regard to things like quality control and automated style of service. In fact, the Golden Arches is known across the Philippines for being quite a stickler when it comes to local affiliates following company guidelines, even going so far as to send out representatives to covertly observe a franchise's daily operations to ensure conformity and quality control.

The franchise for San Fernando's McDonald's was secured by a local ethnic Chinese family whose dealings in municipal commerce date back to the 1930s: the Tans. Although they have operated a number of successful wholesale and retail ventures over the years including the selling of tobacco, groceries, electronics, and appliances, the Tings truly made a name for themselves operating one of the community's most successful commercial firms—the Philippine Bazaar Corporation (PBC).

At the time of its McDonald's franchise acquisition, the PBC's board of directors was comprised of a dozen or so second-generation family members. The firm was officially formed in the early 1980s to consolidate the business holdings created by the first generation of Tan entrepreneurs. By the 1990s, this umbrella company had diversified into a number of specialized trade ventures within the greater San Fernando area. Always on the lookout for new and profitable ventures, a move into the Philippines' growing fast food sector had been something the Tans contemplated for several years.

So it was in the mid-1990s that the family decided to approach McGeorge with an unsolicited proposal to open a McDonald's franchise in San Fernando. The timing of this offer was rather fortuitous considering the Golden Arches in the midst of expanding its corporate footprint in northern Luzon (Philippine Daily Inquirer 1998). To further expedite matters, the firm had something of an inside track for securing this partnership since the wife of McGeorge CEO George Yang, Kristine, was related by marriage to one of the PCB board members. Such personal ties can arguably make a difference when it comes to securing a profitable franchise opportunity in places like the Philippines.

Despite such favorable conditions, all did not go smoothly for the Tans in the lead-up to the contract finalization. McDonald's prospective franchise agreement for San Fernando was delayed for some time given inefficiencies in the Philippines' system for registering company names. In effect, the PBC had to come up with an original and previously unused company name to complete contract negotiations with McGeorge. After several false-starts, the Tans eventually settled upon the never before used corporate name. With this step now complete, the PBC application met with little resistance from McDonald's representatives. Upon successfully fulfilling the franchise application process, the Tans were approved as restaurant operators in 1996.

One of the things that set the new McDonald's apart from its subsequent competitors was that it did not occupy a space within a previously established commercial building but, rather, operated as a free-standing outlet. Deviating somewhat from the Golden Arches' typical franchise agreements in the Philippines, McGeorge and not the Tans owns the site and building where the McDonald's is located. In terms of products and menu items, all of the ingredients come from McDonald's. The meat, napkins, utensils, and other supplies come from McDonald's. Some of the fresh ingredients like lettuce and other vegetables are provided by local producers. These relationships are established and maintained by McDonald's and not the Tan family.

The new McDonald's also diverges from its main fast food competitors in San Fernando as it is geared mainly for those living or working outside of the *población*. The Tans made a special effort to attract those customers more inclined to make the short trip from downtown: namely, jeepney passengers and people with private vehicles. This orientation toward local commuters is reflected in a number of car-friendly features including a passenger drop-off area, a sizable parking lot, and—for the first time in this part of the Philippines—a drive-thru window.

Having dined there multiple times over the years, I can attest that San Fernando's initial McDonald's restaurant lives up to the efficiency and standards that consumers expect from the fast food giant. Customers are greeted by a life-size Ronald McDonald replica as they enter the premises. The well-lit interior gives the place a family-friendly atmosphere. Beyond food, the restaurant also offers consumers amenities like an indoor playground, children's birthday parties, clean restrooms, and a stylish design. The clientele range from CKC students, families, highway travelers, and foreign tourists to the occasional missionary group.

Approximately 50 workers, all of whom appear youthful and upbeat in their employee uniforms, comprise the restaurant's staff. Like other fast food restaurants in the Philippines, entry-level employees are hired on a contract basis with minimal salaries and almost nothing in the way of benefits. If they perform well, there are opportunities for advancement. Managers often come from outside of the local community. That said, one of the younger Tans served as restaurant manager for a time, even attending McDonald's famous Hamburger University in Oak Brook, Illinois where he learned all aspects of McDonald's operations including how to cook, clean, deal with customers, and dispose of the lard collected in the deep-fryers.

By offering new types of products and services to everyday San Fernandians, McDonald's was able to turn a healthy profit in its first year of operations. So successful was the new McDonald's, in fact, that the Tans soon started plans for another free-standing outlet along the National Highway just north of the *población*. Several downtown properties were considered for this

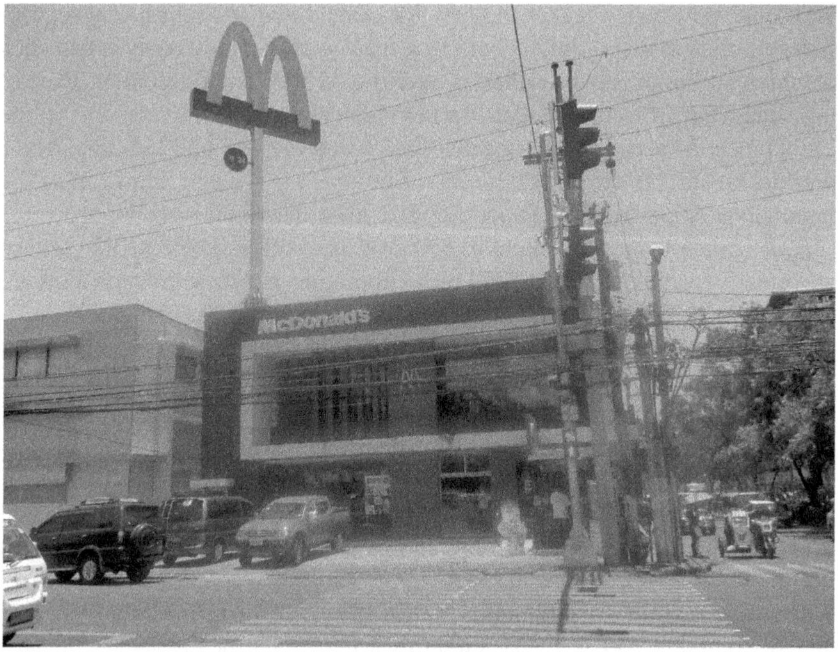


**Figure 3.2 McDonald's, San Fernando City 2015.** Photo taken by Ty Matejowsky.

expansion including the future sites of a second Jollibee restaurant as well as La Union's only KFC branch. The former was bought up at the last minute by Jollibee, while the latter was rejected due to its small size and incompatibility with a drive-thru lane.

It was not until July 2004 that a new McDonald's outlet would open in greater San Fernando City. This more recent venture was housed on the first floor of La Union's first ever shopping mall which is located some three kilometers north of the *población* and operated by the family firm of Dagupan City's current mayor. Since the PBC already had the McDonald's franchise for San Fernando, the Tans were given priority for the new shopping mall McDonald's. Like its counterpart on the National Highway, the mall eatery is not really within walking distance from downtown. Unlike its older sister operation, the new McDonald's lacks amenities such as a playground, drive-thru lane, and party room.

When I chatted with one of the second-generation PBC members in 2006, she states that her family's corporation funded the McDonald's franchises but it is the Manila-based McGeorge that dictates how they run and/or operate both quick-service eateries. She acknowledges that Jollibee was more preferred among Filipinos than McDonald's. To her, the Golden Arches' second place status hinges primarily on the way locals perceive the two competitors' respective menu items. She believes that McDonald's food is viewed as "soggy," while Jollibee fairly is seen as "crispy" and "looking bigger." She states this is because Jollibee uses more flour on their fried chicken batter and hamburger buns to make them appear larger. She says this difference is also notable between Jollibee and KFC.

When I tell her how in the United States customers at McDonald's can now fill and refill their own drinks, she says this would not work in the Philippines because most Filipinos would want to "play" with it. Also, according to her, the reason napkins, utensils, and condiments are doled out at the counter one by one instead of through a self-service format is that most Filipinos would take more than is needed because these items would be perceived as "free." Such sentiments tend to align with those of the other fast food operators and consumers with whom I have chatted.

## JOLLIBEE—SAN FERNANDO CITY (1990s–2010s)

The largest and most popular chain restaurant to open in San Fernando in 1997 was the bi-level Jollibee located in a building complex directly across Quezon Avenue from the town plaza. The spacious eatery sports a yellow/orange/red color scheme with numerous images of the corporate mascot and the slogan "*Langhap Sarap*!" ("Smells Delicious!"). Just outside the first floor entrance, one finds a row of delivery scooters crowded within the narrow parking area where private vehicles compete for access. Since this is the only entry into the restaurant, supplies are regularly transported through the eatery's double doors across the dining area and into a storage room located in back.

Inside, one finds a bustling eatery filled with customers. The lines to the service counter often extend as far back as the store's entrance during busy mealtimes. The upstairs features a playground, banquet room, and restrooms. At almost all hours of the business day, San Fernando's inaugural Jollibee hums with a palpable energy. A steady stream of Western and Tagalog pop music, coupled with the gear-grinding clamor of downtown traffic, adds to the overall vibe of this boisterous atmosphere. It is only in the early morning when customers dine on breakfast items like pancakes, eggs, and *longganisa* that this lively ambience lessens in intensity and become more subdued.

The Jollibee staff is comprised mainly of wage-earners in their late teens and early 20s who offer diners a high level of customer service. While their training expedites the completion of orders in a timely and friendly manner, it sometimes comes up short when encountering situations that veer away from familiar over-the-counter interactions. Like other fast food employees in the Philippines, workers at this particular Jollibee can become flummoxed by unconventional requests.

For instance, in July 2005, I stopped into this Jollibee for a milkshake. After purchasing the frozen dessert, I asked one of the counter staff employees for a delivery menu. From the look on her face it was immediately apparent that she was not prepared to comply with my request. She conferred with a senior employee who in turn told me she would ask the manager. This precipitated a long search for the restaurant manager in the kitchen. When he arrived he politely asked how he could help me. I told him that I would like a menu for take-out/delivery. He informed me that paper menus were never issued to customers. Again, this entire interaction underscores how corporate fast food's "iron cage" can work to fluster employees when confronted with questions or requests that depart from the everyday customer script.

Unlike the new McDonald's, the downtown Jollibee was launched as a branch outlet operated exclusively by the company. For Jollibee, the prospect of minimizing financial risks by taking on a local partner was not a major concern in light of San Fernando's burgeoning fast food scene. The bi-level restaurant features a number of innovations designed with local families in mind. The eatery boasts an indoor playground and rents sections of the second floor for children's birthday parties and other festivities. The company is also a major supporter of local youth events. At area schools or sporting events, the Jollibee mascot often makes an appearance. No less integral to Jollibee's success in San Fernando is its free take-out service. The restaurant employs a number of uniformed drivers to deliver food orders throughout the city via motor scooters. This offering has made the eatery especially popular with downtown professionals who are unable to leave the office during lunch hours.

So well received was Jollibee on the municipal level, in fact, that by 1997 the company bought one of the *población*'s few remaining large commercial lots. Located only three blocks north of its flagship restaurant at a major downtown intersection, the new Jollibee site serves as a multi-branch fast food complex. It houses both another Jollibee as well as an outlet of its sister operation, the company-owned Greenwich Pizza. Over the years the short distance between the two Jollibee restaurants came to include competing chains such as Pizza Hut and KFC. These latter two eateries followed in Jollibee's lead as they were established not as franchises but company-owned branch outlets.

## CHOWKING—SAN FERNANDO CITY (1990s–2010s)

Not enjoying the same level of popularity among San Fernandians as Jollibee or even McDonald's, though still well-liked among diners, is the local

Chowking. The restaurant presents an alternative to the traditional fast food standbys of hamburgers, French fries, and fried chicken by offering selections of Filipino-inspired Chinese cuisine. Consumers can select from a diverse range of menu offerings including *mami* noodles, *siopao* (steamed bun filled with meat), chicken and beef dishes served with rice, and select dessert items.

The chain eatery is the brainchild of Chinese-Filipino Robert F. Kuan, who entered the nation's fast food industry in 1985. Before its acquisition by Jollibee in 2000, his Chowking Foods Corporation had some 130 outlets (5,000 employees) in the Philippines (Quimpo-Espino 1998). By 2015, this number had grown to over 300 branches countrywide with dozens of overseas outlets including several in California and one in Las Vegas, Nevada.

San Fernando's first ever Chowking was established in early 1997 not far from the new Jollibee within a downtown vendor complex known as the Perez Galleria. The local franchise was secured by Raymond and Eduardo Perez, two brothers from a prominent Filipino family that has been active in area commerce and politics for generations. Like the Tans and PBC, the Perez family maintains various business interests in San Fernando including a bank, regional bus line, appliance store, and movie house. Chowking represented their first foray into the restaurant trade.

Before detailing how Chowking established a presence in San Fernando, it is important to recognize the insights provided by Raymond Perez from our July 2006 conversation. I had interviewed him years before in March 1998 when collecting data for my PhD dissertation. Upon reconnecting, it was fairly obvious he did not remember this prior encounter. In fact, he initially assumed I was there as a representative of the Rotary Club, an American-based service organization that he and his family have been involved with for years. Pleasant and accommodating as most Filipinos within this more privileged echelon of society are, he invited me back the following day for a sit-down meeting right around *merienda* time. This arrangement suited me just fine as it gave me ample time to review and refine some of the questions I hoped to ask about his Chowking operations.

The circumstances behind how the Perez brothers secured the Chowking franchise owe as much to serendipity as it does to their business prowess. In the mid-1990s, Raymond was looking for a franchise venture of some kind to occupy the unused sections of the movie theater's lobby. At this point, he was not thinking specifically in terms of fast food. If anything, he wanted something in place to capitalize on this vacant retail space. While he had some previous experience with enterprises of this type—he secured the franchise for Mr. Quickee (a nationwide key and shoe repair company) in San Fernando since 1994—he was not having much success tracking down other franchise opportunities. Things changed in 1996, however, when one of Raymond's film distributors put him in touch with the Manila-based Chowking Food Corporation.

Having dealt with Chowking on previous occasions, the film distributor, without Raymond's knowledge, suggested that company representatives travel to San Fernando to informally inspect the theater lobby. Pleased with what they saw, Chowking offered Raymond a franchise contract almost immediately. At the time, the standard Chowking franchise contract was for ten years and required a capital investment on the part of the franchise holder of approximately ₱8 million with an annual royalty fee of 6 percent of gross sales. Despite such outlays, what made the deal tempting for Raymond was the fact that the restaurant's overhead would remain minimal since he already owned the store property.

If anything was holding Raymond back from pursuing the Chowking franchise, it was the difficulty of meeting all of the franchise expenses on such short notice. Unable to raise the necessary start-up capital alone, especially within a compressed timeframe, he opted to bring in his brother, Eduardo, as the restaurant's primary financial backer. This partnership rendered the prospects of a local Chowking in downtown San Fernando all the more likely. Once the Perez brothers' had their finances in order, the deal moved toward finalization. With construction on the restaurant completed by late 1996, the San Fernando Chowking was ready for its official grand opening in early 1997.

Although the restaurant is smaller and employs fewer workers relative to Jollibee and McDonald's, it does sport many of the same amenities as its rivals including a modern interior design and efficient service system. Tables and chairs are sleek with polished metal touches. On the wall are various prints featuring Chinese characters representing Metal, Water, Wood, Fire, and Earth. A series of footprints leading up to the service counter are traced onto the floor. Diners stand on these outlined imprints as they wait to place their orders. When those up front leave to find seating, everyone else in line moves forward to the next allotted pair of stenciled feet. Rather ingeniously, this subtle method of crowd control expedites the flow of diners and keeps customer queues orderly and untangled.

At dinnertime, the restaurant's 120 seating capacity is usually packed. Patrons select their food items from a backlit menu board that features photos of Chowking dishes with corresponding numbers. Once this transaction is completed, a counter employee announces the orders to the kitchen using the kind of wireless microphone normally reserved for karaoke bars. Diners are then issued a plastic number that is placed on the table while they wait. Within a few minutes, a restaurant employee brings out the food orders. Different from Jollibee and McDonald's, dishes at Chowking are not delivered all at once but whenever they are individually ready. This practice can make for some awkwardness when dining with several friends or co-workers.

Unlike other fast food restaurants in this part of the Philippines, San Fernando's Chowking also features a small corner room that resembles a cross between a religious shrine and museum display. Behind a large ice cream cooler and wall of tinted glass sits a diorama comprised of a wishing well festooned with topiary vines, white Christmas lights, and a statue of St. Vincent Ferrer. Raymond says the display is there to bring good luck. He claims there is an old Filipino folk belief about good luck entailing "not covering the well up to the roof." In this way, the restaurant display really does feature a functioning well. Considering it has an open-air shaft that goes all the way to the roof, a transparent piece of plastic covers the well on rainy days. St. Vincent Ferrer is one of the Catholic saints to which Raymond's mother regularly prays. While he does not really believe in the well's good fortune, he sees it as a way to honor his mother's deeply held religious beliefs. In fact, Raymond has a statue of his own personal saint located on the Perez Galleria's second floor near the movie theater entrance.

At the time of its 1997 launch, Chowking was one of the *población*'s few all-night eateries. Its extended hours attract a pool of customers not usually served by its fast food competitors. The restaurant's late-night clientele include jeepney drivers, movie patrons, and those disembarking or arriving from the nearby bus depot. Despite its popularity with local night owls, according to Raymond, his most loyal customers are not people from San Fernando but rather those who work from 9 to 5 Monday through Friday in downtown. As the administrative center for Region One, San Fernando has numerous offices of government agencies within the city proper. Civil servants that are employed in these departments but live in surrounding communities comprise the bulk of Chowking's patronage. Accordingly, the restaurant's peak business hours coincide with weekday lunch and *merienda* time. "Without these (government) workers," Raymond states, "fast food in San Fernando would die."

On Saturdays and Sundays, Raymond notes an appreciable drop in clientele. So large are the workaday lunchtime crowds, in fact, that Chowking eventually had to expand its dining area to an adjacent space of the Perez Galleria to handle additional weekday customers. This move was done to accommodate consumer overflows as well as to keep patrons from dining elsewhere. The additional room also serves as a function room where various local organizations can hold meetings and seminars. The room is pretty much closed the rest of the time.

Perhaps more distinguishing in the case of Chowking compared to its rivals is its specialized Chinese menu. Chowking offers consumers fast food they cannot get at McDonald's or Jollibee. Especially popular with patrons is *halo-halo*, a decidedly non-Chinese (read Filipino) layered dessert comprised of equal parts of ice cream, condensed milk, crushed ice, diced gelatin, and an assortment of candied toppings. This traditional treat is often consumed at *merienda* and remains one of Chowking's most popular offerings, especially in the summertime when this frozen treat provides welcome relief to the oppressive heat. Although not initially a fan of this ice cream–based dish given its lack of consistent texture, over the years I came to appreciate the frozen dessert's unique character. So much so that I always purchase *halo-halo* whenever I visit Chowking.

Surprisingly, Chowking's main competition does not come from other fast food brands like Jollibee and McDonald's. Rather, it is those local family-owned Chinese restaurants operating in downtown San Fernando that represents the chain's biggest rivals. In fact, Raymond says that since Chowking arrived in 1997 these local ethnic eateries have made slight to significant menu changes to better resemble Chowking fare. For instance, many of these sit-down Chinese restaurants now add sugar to their *siopaos* to be more like the sweet tasting dish served at Chowking. He claims that many local restaurateurs come into Chowking just to keep tabs on the competition.

Raymond and Eduardo hired a Director-in-Charge to oversee their daily interests in the Chowking franchise. Their decision to delegate responsibilities to a salaried supervisor who reported to them exclusively primarily hinged on the fact that, at the time, they had various other business interests to consider and practically no experience running a quick-service eatery. The Director-in-Charge and sometimes Eduardo meet with Chowking representatives on a monthly basis to discuss business strategies and ways to improve sales. The Director-in-Charge also works as a counterpart to the store managers who incidentally are provided by the chain and report goings-on to company representatives back in Manila.

In terms of operations, work duties are handled by two shifts of around 30 total employees. Besides the Director-in-Charge, restaurant personnel include counter staff, cooks, security guards, store managers, and custodial workers. Hiring for all new positions is a rather simple and straightforward process. Ads are posted in the restaurant window for potential employees to see. Once the application period ends, a shortlist of viable candidates is interviewed by the Director-in-Charge and store managers based in part on the data information sheets (i.e., résumés) they provide.

Most entry-level positions are approved by Raymond and Eduardo without the direct consultation of the Chowking Company headquartered in Metro-Manila. Considering most job-seekers are local teenagers and college-age adults, crew members are paid minimum wage and only employed for five-month stints. Short-term contracts like this are the standard in the Philippines' fast food industry as they represent a cost-saving measure to keep employers from providing healthcare and other benefits.

Besides restaurant managers, only head cooks are kept for longer than five months at San Fernando's Chowking. Extended contracts of this sort, however, were not always the norm. According to Raymond, cooks were initially terminated after only five months' service just like other crew members to streamline costs. Such employment policies changed, however, once customers began noticing inconsistencies in the taste and texture of restaurant food. A high kitchen turnover made it difficult to maintain familiar tasting menu items for any significant period of time. Recognizing that such variation could lead diners elsewhere, the Perez brothers began offering cooks more job security as a way to preserve a more standardized and predictable bill of fare from week to week and month to month.

Such tweaks to restaurant operations illustrate the kind of sway Raymond and Eduardo are able to exert over their Chowking franchise even as the company set the parameters for how the chain's eateries are supposed to be run. Raymond says Chowking is open to suggestions from their franchisees. In many cases, the new strategies, innovations, and marketing techniques developed by local affiliates are disseminated at the annual franchise holder conventions that Chowking sponsors. For the most part, such meetings are attended by both franchisees and store managers.

As franchise holders, the Perez brothers are primarily in charge of local marketing and financial support while the company provides the store managers and stationary and seasonal bill of fare. Most of their interactions with the Chowking Company take place through the store managers, who answer partly to the franchise holder but mostly to the corporate office. In fact, restaurant managers provide daily reports to the company. Such information is not always taken at face-value. In some instances, goings-on at restaurants are verified by Chowking representatives who conduct secret on-site inspections to make sure local franchise operations are adhering to corporate policies and practices.

The Perez brothers' franchise agreement with Chowking was finalized some three years before the Chinese restaurant's 2000 acquisition by Jollibee. In the time since, Raymond has noticed modest to significant improvements in chain operations. For one thing, Chowking's corporate look was upgraded. As it became a vital part of the Jollibee family, its color scheme was subtly altered to better compliment the iconic orange, red, and yellow of the Philippines top fast food brand. Today, Chowking advertising and storefronts feature a combination of red, blue, white, and apricot. More significantly, Jollibee introduced a lighted picture menu board as a part of its subsidiary's restaurant operations. This addition increased efficiency at the counter as customers now only have to look and point to their order. Prior to this time, counter staff often spent considerable time describing the look and ingredient of everyday menu items. This improvement expedited counter transactions and customer flows began to move more efficiently.

Like their Jollibee and McDonald's rivals, the 2004 launch of a new shopping mall in San Fernando City's urban periphery proved a cause for concern to the Perez brothers. Questions arose about how this new consumer facility with its various fast food offerings would impact established dining patterns and retail trade in the *población*. Raymond thinks many downtown businesses took a hit when the mall first opened but over time were able to recover. As of 2006, he says local consumers are split between downtown and the mall; stating that many prefer the latter as a weekend hangout. He and Eduardo even mulled the possibility of opening another Chowking outlet in the new shopping center but quickly reconsidered since the only available spot featured an unsuitable location and pricey monthly rental fee. Based on their projections at the time, a potential mall Chowking would be lucky to break even under these circumstances. He says there was a Shakey's Pizza outlet near the plaza that shut down to relocate inside the mall.

## DAGUPAN VERSUS SAN FERNANDO CITY

Besides a few select differences, the penetration of corporate fast food into Dagupan and beginning in the 1980s resembles events in San Fernando City in most key ways. Quick-service eateries in both communities were launched either through (1) franchising agreements between chains headquartered in Metro-Manila and local entrepreneurs or through (2) national and international brands establishing their own company-run branch outlets. As discussed in chapter 2, franchising represents a viable option for fast food brands looking to minimize some of the financial risks associated with launching a venture at the community level.

Similarly, like developments in Dagupan City, those in San Fernando followed a nearly identical pattern whereby American-style fast food restaurants first appeared in and around the *población* before spreading to more peripheral areas. Almost invariably, this commercial expansion paralleled the rise of modern shopping malls located beyond the traditional downtown cores of urban commerce. In fact, these modern consumer venues helped expedite growth in the number and selection of local fast food chains.

Finally, the growth of corporate fast food in both Dagupan and San Fernando exhibited distinctive ethnic dimensions wherein a small number of minority-owned trade firms actively lead the establishment of this particular style of dining. With the notable exclusion of Chowking in San Fernando, most of the restaurant ventures examined in this chapter were spearheaded by Chinese-Filipino families with longstanding roots in urban commerce.

Considering that the national franchises for most of the Philippines' top homegrown and global fast food chains are held by Chinese-Filipinos, such occurrences in Dagupan and San Fernando are not entirely surprising.

When considered in tandem, Dagupan and San Fernando City's respective experiences with American-style quick-service eateries challenge certain notions about corporate fast food's global hegemony. The opening of a few small downtown outlets followed by the launch of more conspicuous brands like McDonald's, Jollibee, and Chowking in and around the cities' *poblacións* starting in the 1990s effectively counters prevailing narratives whereby local interests remain all but excluded from processes of fast food market growth. Rather than serving as passive bystanders in this unfolding expansion, key groups and individuals in both communities actively abet the spread of this dining format into heretofore untapped provincial areas.

If the experiences of Dagupan and San Fernando City offer any indication, local interests have emerged as viable partners in corporate fast food's global advancement that suggest both a receptiveness and willingness to engage this ostensibly homogenizing dining format. In the most conspicuous of ways, local involvement in such developments takes the form of capital investment and/or retail partnerships with Manila-based chains. These national operations have a discernible effect in Dagupan, San Fernando, and other Philippine towns and cities on how fast food production and consumption is ultimately expressed in municipal commerce. Such impacts are manifested primarily through the indigenization of menu items to better conform to Filipino palates. The aforementioned mango shakes (Jollibee), McSpaghetti (McDonald's), and *halo-halo* (Chowking) demonstrate such tendencies. Within the franchises themselves, the efforts of local owner-operators to alter or change aspects of their restaurant operations typically occur within the sometimes narrow parameters implemented from above. Even as Manila-based chains impose constraints on how restaurants operate, findings from both cities reveal some degree of agency on the part of local entrepreneurs that work to indigenize or reshape manifestations of corporate fast food at the community level. Perhaps nowhere is this more apparent than the Perez brothers' Chowking operations in San Fernando City.

In the next chapter—following a personal vignette culled from my 2015 Dagupan City fieldnotes—I examine the various ways top fast food companies work to attract and retain a devoted following of preschool, teen, and preadolescent diners. Thus, a primary focus of chapter 4 is the methods Jollibee, McDonald's, and other popular chains employ to entice young Filipino audiences both directly and indirectly. Findings in this section draw heavily from my own ethnographic research in Dagupan and San Fernando City dating back to the 1990s as well as several different secondary sources. In fact, I include the near word-for-word fieldnotes I compiled after participating in a

2006 Jollibee children's birthday party. The subsequent portrait that emerges reveals just how much capital and coordinated effort established restaurant chains invest in securing and expanding the patronage of successive generations of loyal customers.

Cutting across diverse marketing and media platforms, the fast food industry's ability to reach this impressionable demographic appears almost as sophisticated as it does efficacious. While the multi-pronged approaches adopted by top quick-service eateries in the Philippines are in many ways comparable to those currently encountered in North America and Europe, in other respects they exhibit notable differences. In some cases, the promotional efforts of McDonald's and Jollibee in today's Philippines are not unlike those previously aimed at Western preschool and school-age kids some years back.

Due to growing concerns about the ill-effects of fast food marketing directed at children voiced by parents and public health advocates in North America and elsewhere, however, these one-time practices were eventually retooled or phased out entirely. Indeed, those familiar staples of Happy Meals from yesteryear such as salty French fries and sugary sodas have been replaced in the United States with the more healthy options of apple slices and low-fat milk. Since industry efforts of this variety still remain largely muted in the Philippines, the next chapter offers some revealing insights into a national fast food scene that is arguably more expansive, if not slightly more tolerant, when it comes to the particular influence corporate fast food exerts over young people.

# Chapter 4

# The Young and the Hungry

## *Fast Food and Children 2000s–2010s*

### VIGNETTE TWO: A PERSONAL ACCOUNT FROM THE FIELD, MCDONALD'S, DAGUPAN CITY, PANGASINAN, FRIDAY, MAY 15, 2016, EARLY MORNING

It never seems to fail but at some point during my visits to the Philippines I grow weary of local fare and begin craving the more familiar tastes of home. Right or wrong, I have traveled here often enough to feel little shame about indulging this desire for the brands and products that reflect the mainstream sensibilities of American consumers.

While the presence of U.S. chains overseas is easy to decry as some abstract menace eroding cultural heterogeneity worldwide, such attitudes can easily soften when confronted by a profound appetite for the familiar. Doubtless this is something I hesitate admitting in anthropological circles where a sophisticated and adventurous palate is as esteemed as prevailing theoretical bents. Yet, if I am being honest with myself, acknowledging this predilection is essential for understanding how much my consumption choices abroad are influenced by utilitarian considerations of convenience, familiarity, and taste and how much they are, perhaps unconsciously, driven by brand appeal and marketing.

So it is during this current visit to Dagupan City, after back-to-back mornings of mostly stale instant coffee packaged in single serving sachets and heated up in my hotel room with mostly tepid results, I find myself seized by an intense, almost visceral, desire for some freshly brewed Starbucks coffee. Departing my hotel along the Pantal River, I head west down A. B. Fernandez Avenue toward the gleaming new coffeehouse that, according to the desk clerk, opened a few months back.

It is not yet 7 am and the powerful longing for good java grips my consciousness with surprising severity. More than just a little chagrined about my current predicament, I nevertheless recognize the need to address the situation head-on lest I suffer further irritability, intestinal irregularity, and other unenviable consequences of what feels like prolonged coffee deprivation. Knowing that relief is only a few blocks away, I anxiously anticipate the life-affirming jolt of caffeine that helps take the edge off that jittery sense of anxiousness that frays my sensibilities and renders me barely functional.

As I make my way along the city's uneven sidewalks, I cannot help but notice just how sparse downtown traffic is at this early hour. Few shops are open for business; most remain hidden behind solid metal gates that roll down from above to secure storefront entrances and safeguard the merchandise contained therein. With the exception of a stray jogger or overnight security guard killing time before the next shift arrives, the business district appears nearly deserted. It is at times like these that Dagupan City exhibits an eerie kind of tranquility that throws the bustling tempo of workaday street life into stark relief.

Looming in the distance I make out the unmistakable contours of the city's first modern shopping mall which extend well above the rooflines of adjacent low- and mid-rise buildings. Constructed over 20 years ago, it stands on the original site of the municipal public marketplace which partially collapsed during the 1990 earthquake. At the time of its 1994 opening, the new retail complex was touted by many as irrefutable proof that downtown Dagupan had at last moved beyond the disaster's profound devastation. Considering it was the first major consumer venue of its kind, north of Metro-Manila, the mall did much to revitalize local commerce, attracting customers from around Pangasinan and beyond. In no small way, it showed that commercial centers of this variety were a viable investment for developers looking to expand into provincial markets.

Over the years, as new and larger shopping malls commenced operations in the urban periphery and neighboring towns, this once-thriving venture slowly fell into disrepair and out of favor with local shoppers. Notwithstanding recent efforts to revitalize its flagging image, the downtown mall now retains little of its former vibrancy. On the outside, the unrelenting tropical sun has leached away much of the mall's once vivid pink and aqua color scheme. On the inside, few of the original chain clothing and electronic stores from 1994 remain in business. Most have been replaced with small mom and pop vending operations that are effectively identical to those found in the nearby public marketplace.

To say that this mall has seen better days is probably no great exaggeration. Yet, even as numerous shops have come and gone over the years, the McDonald's and Shakey's Pizza that bookend the mall's main entrance exhibit a kind of staying power that eludes most other first floor occupants.

These chain eateries have lost little of their popular appeal, representing some of the only tenants that have maintained a continuous presence here since 1994. In fact, the Golden Arches sign that towers above the mall parking lot and nearby city hall has become a fixture of downtown's skyline for some two decades now.

After passing under a soot-smudged pedestrian flyover, I weave through some vehicles parked catty-corner to an unopened bank with a roof billboard promoting the recent Mayweather-Pacquiao prizefight ("The Fight of the Century"). I catch my first glimpse of the upscale coffee shop. The mere sight of the iconic green and white logo, a two-tailed mermaid sporting a crown, is enough to trigger a Pavlovian sense of anticipation somewhere deep inside me. A rick dark roast within the quiet and pleasant surroundings of this familiar coffeehouse beckons. If my coffee craving cannot be more obvious, I move briskly up the steps with alacrity that even the unwieldiness of my backpack cannot impede.

A firm pull on the door pretty much extinguishes all of my enthusiasm. A heavy steel chain and padlock wrapped around the glassed double doors denies me entrance. Peering through the tinted glass for a few moments, I catch the attention of a college-aged employee sporting the familiar black and green hat and apron combo coming out of a back room. He arches his eyebrows and makes an "oh" with his mouth in that very characteristic Filipino gesture before shaking his head and using his puckered lips to point to a sign indicating store business hours. Apparently this Starbucks does not open for another 20 minutes or so. Feeling deflated, I cut across A. B. Fernandez Avenue and park myself on a concrete bench near a grove of palm trees by the city plaza.

When I return to the Starbucks about ten after seven, nothing has seemingly changed except that the store now appears completely devoid of workers. Even with the interior lights off I can still see various pastries, snacks, and bottled juices on display under the refrigerated glass case. I find it curious that even though the Starbucks is situated directly across from city hall no office workers are clamoring to get in.

Discouraged but undeterred, I backtrack to try my luck at the shopping mall McDonalds. Upon entering, I am immediately struck by how much the restaurant has changed since I first ate there in 1994. A more sophisticated and cozy décor that would seem befitting in the nearby Starbucks has replaced the interchangeable tables and booths that once lined the dining space in neat rows. Today, the restaurant's eating area features sleek counters and tabletops, some of which include padded seating or stools sporting red and black accents.

At this early hour the McDonald's is not even half-full. Scattered among the various empty chairs and tables sit a few middle-aged business types, leisurely drinking coffee, casually leafing through newspapers. Near the wash station and glassed party room, a group of coeds stay glued to their mobile phones seemingly uninterested in conversing with one another. The air-conditioning blows languidly, barely cooling the place. Near the service counter, the unmistakable smells of coffee and cooking grease tinge the air. Under different circumstances I would probably find such "greasy spoon" odors slightly off-putting but given my limited prospects for some decent dark roast, they seem to promise the next best thing.

A quick scan of the lighted menu board reveals a familiar selection of breakfast choices that most non-Filipinos can appreciate. Just like in the United States, these items can be purchased individually or as value meals. In most cases this means orders come with sides of coffee and hash browns. Friendly but not particularly chatty, a McDonald's crewmember takes my order for an Egg McMuffin meal by gingerly tapping the surface of a digital touchscreen that faintly illuminates her features in the restaurant's pallid light. She thanks me for paying with exact change before assembling the contents of my order onto a plastic tray.

Moving ostensibly at half-speed, she places a napkin, packets of sugar, dairy creamer, and ketchup on the paper-lined surface one by one. Using a pair of metal thongs, she retrieves a hash brown from the deep-fryer, slides it into a paper sleeve, and deposits it on to the tray. Off to the side, a bespectacled manager uses a pocket calculator to count the contents of a cash drawer. The restaurant's hushed atmosphere makes every keypad punch distinctly audible.

After what seems like several minutes, my tray contains everything but the breakfast sandwich and coffee. I am asked to find a seat and issued a metal table number so that the rest of my order can be brought out momentarily. Perhaps to make up for the delay, the crewmember gives me a free newspaper. Selecting a table near a glassed wall that looks out on the darkened mall, it is clear that McDonald's is the only place open for business at this early hour.

Various tarp-covered kiosks that sell cell phone accessories, plastic kitchenware, and assorted merchandise sit between an out of commission one-way escalator and a set of stairs that ascend upward to the third floor. At some point, a McDonald's radio station that plays an eclectic mix of Tagalog and Western pop hits interspersed with commercials and company jingles is switched on. I recognize songs by Sheryl Crow, the Goo Goo Dolls, and Keane but some of those from Asian performers fail to register. Later, I note a stripped-down version of Foster the People's "Pumped Up Kicks" by a Filipina artist whose name I do not catch. The singer's sincere and inoffensive vocal feels notably at odds with song's dark subject matter and lyrics, particularly the line "better run faster than my bullets."

At long last, the McDonald's manager brings out my order. She thanks me for my patience after collecting the metal table number. Between sips and bites of the Egg McMuffin, I retrieve a lined composition book from my backpack and begin jotting down some initial impressions of the eatery and downtown Dagupan. Having learned the hard way about putting off such a simple but vital task, I try to meticulously document everything within my surroundings in case the details slip away later. On my way to the service counter for a refill of coffee a few moments later, I notice a self-service "water and gravy area" off to the side. Two simple dispensers allow customers to self-provision themselves with these side items. I know many fast food diners in the Philippines like to add servings of the warm brown liquid to orders of fried chicken or steamed rice.

Throughout the eatery, paper signs promoting the McFlurry dessert ("Love it to Bits") hang from the ceiling. More numerous are those placards advertising a phone number for free McDonald's delivery. Apparently, customers can text or call in their orders and moped drivers will transport their food purchases to residential or work addresses throughout the city. The digits for this service even appear printed on receipts and McDonald's sugar packets.

I enjoy a second coffee as a fly buzzes around my wrapper-strewn tray. The Egg McMuffin pretty much like what is offered at McDonald's stateside while the hash brown came out far too greasy for me to sample. I use my composition book to scribble down some tasks I hope to accomplish today. For one, I plan on donating some of my published ethnographic work focusing on Dagupan and Pangasinan to the main city library. Based on past experience, I suspect this gesture will receive a mostly deadpan or inscrutable reaction from staff workers. The rest of the day will be spent lining up interviews and making the rounds to touch base with some old friends and acquaintances.

Sometime after 8 am, a uniformed security guard opens up the shopping center's main entrance to let in a throng of mall employees. They file through in groups and pairs; some clutching plastic bags, some holding hands. Within this crowd, I spot a boy and girl wearing McDonald's caps and shirts walk toward the fast food eatery accompanied by an adult. From the looks of it, the twosome is taking part in some type of restaurant promotional event. They cut across the dining area, sporting red lanyards around their necks, on the way to the glassed-in party room where the female restaurant manager greets them enthusiastically. It is around this time that I notice that the banquet area is festooned with various colorful balloons and streamers. Several employees busily add last-minute touches to these decorations as a children's celebration is presumably about to get under way.

Almost at once, the pace of activity in the McDonald's noticeably shifts into high gear. As more customers arrive, work at the registers and in the kitchen starts to pick up. Pretty soon, restaurant staff is circulating throughout the eatery, attending to tables of students, grandparents with grandkids, and assorted business types. Workers bring out breakfast orders and collect the metal numbers. Some employees begin wiping down tabletops while others discard refuse into metal bins located near the exit doors. Customers eat and talk loudly on their mobile phones or with each other.

Preparing to leave, I observe more kids wearing McDonald's-inspired hats and attire arrive and file into the party room with adults in tow. Seating inside this glassed area now appears at full capacity as the venue pulses with chatter and excitement. About a dozen or so participants sit at tables alongside their adoring parents. I approach an employee in his early twenties conversing with a store security guard in the hopes of finding out more about these goings-on. When I ask him about the children's event, the young man whose name tag reads "Eric" tells me it is a graduation ceremony for a weeklong McDonald's workshop. He calls it the "Kiddie Crew," saying it is held every summer to teach children things like "hard work and teamwork."

With Eric's consent, I slip into the party room to snap a few pictures and just get a better sense of what the "Kiddie Crew" is all about. An awards ceremony is in progress. Kids are brought up one by one to receive a certificate and have their picture taken with various restaurant employees in front of a table loaded with all sorts of McDonald's swag. Presumably, these items will go to the kids once the ceremony wraps up. A few parents shoot curious glances in my direction but most of the attention remains focused on what takes place up front. Not wanting to over stay my welcome, I quickly slide back into the dining area and head toward the exit. Before departing, I stop to thank Eric for accommodating me. As is often the case, he peppers me with a few questions.

"From what country do you come?" asks Eric.

"The U.S."

"Do you work for McDonald's?" he asks.

"No, I'm just interested in fast food. So, what kind of activities do the kids do?"

"They do artwork and even work behind the counter making cheeseburgers."

"Really? That's great. By the way, how are they chosen to participate?"

My query receives no reply. Eric is promptly called away to attend to some minor kitchen emergency or maybe that he just doesn't want to talk anymore. At any rate, I exit the restaurant and make my way through the mall's parking lot. Traffic on A. B. Fernandez Avenue has picked up considerably. Cars, jeepneys, and tricycles tap their brakes, moving haphazardly along the hot asphalt. The morning air becomes redolent with the unmistakable scent of exhaust fumes. A hazy sort of mist starts to tinge everything at street level with discernible nicotine brownness. Using my hand as a makeshift pollution mask to filter out the contaminants, I walk with serious intent not toward the hotel but instead to the Starbucks across the street. I am determined to record everything Eric told me about the "Kiddie Crew" while the details still remain fresh. The coffee shop's proximity, comfortable surroundings, and amenities such as free Wi-Fi make it an ideal setting for firing up my laptop to type some more fieldnotes and search the Internet for more information on the "Kiddie Crew."

## FAST FOOD AND CHILDREN

The contours of day-to-day life in the Philippines have undergone varying degrees of reconfiguration over the past 35 years thanks in part to the far-reaching influence of corporate fast food. The successful inroads made by national and multinational chain restaurants at the community level have steadily transformed aspects of Philippine society, especially those related to local foodways and dietary habits. Similarly, my own research in Dagupan City, Pangasinan reveals that nearly 90 percent of 161 surveyed college students consume fast food cuisine at least once or twice per month (Matejowsky 2008), and only 5 percent characterize its dietary value as nutritionally deficient or unhealthy (Matejowsky 2009). While these findings may raise serious concerns for healthcare professionals, nutritionists, and policymakers as obesity and obesity-related conditions intensify nationwide and globally (Mydans 2003; Popkin 2008), they also highlight just how far corporate fast food has taken root within the sociocultural schema of today's Philippines (Conde 2005).

As I have previously argued here and elsewhere (Matejowsky 2006; 2007; 2008; 2009), the multifarious effect of Western-style fast food on Philippine life now effectively transcends matters of food production and consumption. Corporate fast food plays an increasingly influential role in (re)shaping the consumer sensibilities, social lives, consumption practices, nationalist sentiments, and, significantly, childhood experiences of most moderate and less affluent Filipinos (Matejowsky 2006:146; Matejowsky 2008).

An examination of the country's vibrant fast food scene reveals many of the historical nuances and interrelated social, political, and economic processes that presently define Philippine modernity. The complexities underlying the spread of quick-service eateries throughout the Visayas, Mindanao, and Luzon provide a viable context for understanding the various ambivalences informing Filipino views about postcolonialism and American society (Matejowsky 2007). Moreover, they also illuminate an emerging neo-patriotism that is subtly expressed through local consumption practices and brand preferences, particularly amid the ongoing rivalry between global pioneer McDonald's and the more highly profitable and popular indigenous chain, Jollibee (Matejowsky 2008).

As in other countries of East and Southeast Asia, the fast food industry has gone to great lengths to attract and maintain a wide following of repeat customers in the Philippines (Watson 1997). Through targeted marketing campaigns, social media innovations, sleek aesthetics, indigenized menus, and on-site amenities like piped music, air-conditioning, and clean restrooms, McDonald's, Jollibee, and many of their chief competitors have developed a loyal consumer base that continues to patronize local outlets even as the nation's economic performance undergoes periods of fluctuating, if sometimes slack growth. Indeed, the country's thriving fast food sector represents one of the few consistent bright spots of commercial achievement within a historically underperforming domestic marketplace (Matejowsky 2008).

Since the early 1980s, a key aspect of corporate fast food's success in the Philippines has been its orientation of products and operations toward Filipino families and children. The restaurant playgrounds, junior-sized meals with small toys, Hollywood blockbuster promotional tie-ins, and advertising narratives that reflect traditional Filipino values are but a few examples of this now-standard industry approach. Perhaps nothing better exemplifies this child-centric slant within local milieus than the Jollibee corporate mascot's seemingly ubiquitous presence.

Like a decidedly homegrown counterpoint to the Golden Arches' iconic Ronald McDonald, images of this giant cartoon bee with the cherubic face and puffy plumed chef's hat abound in and around the hundreds of Jollibee outlets that dot towns and cities across the archipelago. The highway billboards, restaurant signage, and other representations of the orange, red, and yellow Jollibee logo stand out vividly against the sometimes harsh street-level urban fabric that characterizes most Philippine cityscapes. This outdoor advertising, coupled with an almost incessant stream of Jollibee television, radio, and web commercials, gives the chain a pervasive market presence that at times can feel almost oversaturated.

Given Jollibee's overarching influence nationwide, it is probably not surprising that the corporate mascot has emerged as the country's most widely recognized children's character (Wong 2007). While Ronald McDonald may hold this distinction in other parts of the world, the Philippines again remains one of the few places where the clown's popularity remains subordinate to that of the bee. Manifestations of Jollibee's ongoing favorability among kids and families are expressed in diverse ways in restaurant operations and popular culture.

Indeed, Jollibee's high profile has spawned various subsidiary ventures oriented toward kids including a line of toys, clothing, and a nationally televised half-hour program, *Jollitown*, which began airing in 2007 to commemorate the chain's 30th anniversary. The show bears little resemblance to the retail direct-to-video animated series put out by the Golden Arches in the late 1990s entitled *The Wacky Adventures of Ronald McDonald*. While the McDonald's show was clearly *Rugrats* inspired, *Jollitown* differs in that it features real-life kids interacting with the costumed bee and several secondary Jollibee characters that were introduced to consumers over the years including Yum the Scientist (a hamburger-headed science enthusiast introduced in 1985), Hetty the Cheerleader (a cheerleader with spaghetti locks introduced in 1984), Popo the Gym Coach (a track-suited blonde lad with French-fry hair introduced in 1985), and Twirlie the Star Performer (a sparkly mall chick with a chocolate sundae bouffant introduced in 1988) (Afinidad 2008).

With production values and storylines befitting most children's programming in today's Philippines, weekly episodes depict the amicable goings-on of this imaginary fast food gang. Music, dancing, and lessons of friendship and cooperation are all conveyed against the backdrop of an enchanted fast food village that not so subtly asserts the wholesomeness of Jollibee's brand image.

I actually bought a pirated DVD of the inaugural series as gift for my kids during my summer 2010 fieldwork in San Fernando City. Somewhat coincidentally, I purchased the disc at a vendor kiosk right outside of the second Jollibee constructed in downtown. Wrapped in cheap cellophane and a crudely photoshopped paper sleeve, the program became an unexpected household hit for several weeks upon my return home. My sons and daughter were transfixed by the almost surreal depictions of brightly costumed characters interacting with child actors in the titular *Jollitown*, a fast food village created almost entirely through computer-generated imagery and green screen technology. While the Jollibee character narrates on-screen happenings in both English and Tagalog, a repetitive kind of background music plays on a loop. In more than one way, *Jollitown* owes as much to the campy sensibilities of kid television favorites such as the *Power Rangers* or Sid and Marty Kroft productions from the 1970s as it does the simple minimalist production of the *Teletubbies*.

*Jollitown* was broadcast for several seasons each Sunday morning in this original format on the GMA Network before moving to rival channel ABS-CBN where it was aired on Saturdays as *The Jollitown Kids Show*. In either iteration, the show was classified as educational programming even though it was basically a half-hour-long advertisement for Jollibee and Jollibee products. Perhaps its educational credentials were most in evidence in season five which focused primarily on important events in Philippine history. Suffice it to say, the show did much to burnish the chain's image among youngsters and reinforce the cartoon bee's near ubiquity across the islands.

## FAST FOOD CONSUMPTION, KIDS MEALS, AND TOYS

As one might expect, Filipinos like their American counterparts begin eating fast food at a young age. Findings from my 2005 survey of 161 undergraduate Dagupeños provide some suggestion of when Filipinos first start consuming fast food. Some 45 percent (73 students) of those responding report originally trying this style of cuisine between the ages of one and five years old. Twenty-eight percent (45 students) report being between six and ten years old, while approximately 18 percent (29 students) were between 11 and 15 years old. Without overestimating these survey data's relevance, they do offer select indication of just how young Filipinos are when they begin eating this type of fare.

Efforts to reach and retain such young audiences by Jollibee, McDonald's, and others in the Philippines' fast food industry extend beyond television programs and demographically focused advertising. After the Golden Arches introduced Filipinos to its iconic small-serving-boxed meal, the Happy Meal, in 1997, other national and international brands followed suit. Indeed, rare is the quick-service chain that does not offer some kind of kids' dining option that includes giveaways like small toys or promotional tie-ins with the latest hit movie or cartoon series. While these mass-produced items are not really known for their durability or status as irreplaceable keepsakes, they do serve as an added inducement for children looking to convince their parents or grandparents to treat them to a fast food meal. As in the United States, these disposable toys, games, and related novelties are usually only offered for a limited time or while supplies last with new toy lines rotating in every few weeks.

In certain cases and doubtless to the delight of that certain breed of fanboy who scours the World Wide Web looking for the latest movie marketing oddity that dramatically misses the mark, these promotional tie-ins can sometimes live on in infamy due to the unintended consequences of poor design or conceptual miscalculation. Such was the case in 2012 when Jollibee won the right to promote a reboot of the global blockbuster franchise *The Amazing Spiderman* in the Philippines. What drew its fair share of online sniggers was not the inclusion of a small slingshot that allowed kids to fling tiny projectiles at a paper likeness of The Lizard villain nor the compact red and blue LED projector but rather the plastic ring-toss game that came with the purchase of buckets of Jollibee's signature fried chicken product, Chicken-joy. Indeed, the wall-crawling superhero's perch atop a pyramid of frozen webbing triggered guffaws across the Internet as it gave the anatomically suspect impression of a "rectal violation of the web slinger" (Slager 2012).

The Jollibee and McDonald's restaurants that I frequented in San Fernando and Dagupan over the years typically displayed these knickknacks either in storefront windows or in colorful showcases near the service counter and well within the sightline of young diners. Even as a kid, promotions of this sort never really appealed to me but on one occasion in 2005 they did produce their desired effect. That summer, I bought several Jollibee Kiddiee Meals not so much for the hamburgers and French fries but rather for the *Star Wars: Revenge of the Sith* items that were included with purchase. These toys were ostensibly for my children but if truth be told were actually for me. This collection of inexpensive sci-fi toys and gadgets included various well-known characters from the *Star Wars* prequels including a prized R2-D2 facsimile lunchbox that I still have somewhere wrapped in its original packaging.

Clearly, offerings of this variety are not all that different from standard fast food practices and promotions in North America and elsewhere. Perhaps more so than other non-Western populations, Filipinos remain well attuned to the popular personalities, products, and lifestyles disseminated by the U.S. cultural industry every year, including those celebrated movies, television shows, comics, and other child-centric media showcased as promotional tie-ins with kid-sized meals. Most Westerners would doubtless recognize, although not necessarily condone, such marketing efforts in the Philippines as they are aimed directly at the impressionable minds of young children.

In fact, even as there has been a recent push across North America and Europe to severely restrict or modify this kind of advertising given its associations with rising obesity and ill-health, such activism has not yet taken root elsewhere. The fact that the Philippines lacks any major consumer advocacy group to raise, much less sustain, awareness about the deleterious effects of diets based around fast food and other fatty, calorically dense, and sodium-rich products makes industry practices of this sort all the more problematic. Perhaps a first step in tamping down any burgeoning local criticism in the Philippines is McDonald's decision to donate a small amount of its proceeds from every Happy Meal sold to various charities including its own Ronald McDonald House which hosts families with children undergoing intensive hospital care. Until such time that public sentiments shift away from ostensible indifference or tacit approval of targeted restaurant promotions like this, toys will surely remain essential components of both kids' fast food meals and industry efforts at building customer loyalty and brand equity among young audiences.

## KIDDIE CREW AND KIDS CLUB

The preceding examples do not deviate much from child-centric fast food practices observed elsewhere. Indeed, what kid growing up in the United States since the 1980s has not consumed their fair share of Happy Meals or at the very least been exposed to the marketing allure of fast food and its associated promotional toys or tie-ins? That said, there are areas where attempts at attracting and engaging a kid clientele by quick-service eateries in the Philippines differ slightly to significantly with the methods employed by their North American and European counterparts.

In what would surely spark criticism from Western consumers and parents given the ongoing controversies surrounding health and labor issues related to corporate fast food in the United States, Canada, and Europe, both McDonald's and Jollibee sponsor a specialized form of fast food outreach designed to directly connect with school-aged children. Unlike the kind of restaurant fan clubs or promotional efforts whereby enrollees receive a membership card, some sort of modest prize, or discount on menu items, these more exclusive initiatives offer participants an immersive hands-on fast food experience that arguably blurs the line between a fun-filled summer activity and new employee training.

McDonald's "Kiddie Crew Workshop" and Jollibee's "Kids Club Talent Camp" are popular promotions geared specifically toward the sensibilities of boys and girls aged six through twelve. For several weeks each summer both chains hold these weekday workshops—actually more like day camps—at hundreds of restaurant locations nationwide. Rather than compete with regular diners for sometimes scarce seating, campers are typically sequestered off from other patrons in the restaurant party room. Since their respective launches in the 1990s, thousands of Filipino youth have completed these programs.

Like other daytime activities designed to keep children occupied when school is not in session, the "Kiddie Crew Workshop" and "Kids Club Talent Camp" combine all types of arts and crafts and fun and games with lessons that promote both positive social values and experiential learning. Sometimes obviously, sometimes less so, these respective offerings can appear to casual observers as little more than the first step toward a successful fast food career. Considering participants receive real on-the-floor training that entails things like working the register, making their own burgers, and filling customer orders at the service counter and drive-thru lane, such impressions are difficult to deny.

Enrollment in the McDonald's "Kiddie Crew Workshop" goes for around ₱600 ($13) per child. Since this effectively prices out most ordinary families, campers tend to come from affluent or modestly well-off households. The registration fee not only offsets expenses related to the various promotional items participants receive (t-shirts, hats, bags, art supplies, and completion certificates), it also covers the cost of meals for five days. For a few hours each morning, Crew participants get to learn new company-inspired songs (the "Kiddie Crew Theme") and dances ("Do-the-Ronald") as well as complete assorted art and cooking projects. These activities include things such as making their own aprons, designing Happy Meal boxes, and preparing hamburgers

On the company website and promotional materials, the day camp is presented, in part, as a venue for instilling important values. Kids learn the importance of principles like teamwork, handiwork, responsibility, discipline, and sharing through lectures given by McDonald's managers. At the end of the week, Crew members are not only treated to a graduation ceremony where diplomas and all variety of McDonald's swag are awarded, they also get to perform to their parents and other audience members the songs and dances they have learned over the previous days.

Never one to tamper with a proven formula, Jollibee pretty much co-opted McDonald's approach to directly engaging Filipino youngsters in this way when it unveiled its own take on the kids' workshop concept some years after the Golden Arches. Notwithstanding some minor variations in camp duration and activities, the homegrown chain gives its enrollees a fast food experience nearly identical to the one offered by its main competitor. The "Kids Club Talent Camp" basically mirrors McDonald's "Kiddie Crew" in that it features a curriculum of activities where kids create simple Jollibee-themed handicrafts, choreography, skits, and songs in addition to crafting their own hamburgers.

Like McDonald's, Jollibee campers receive a commemorative t-shirt and assorted keepsakes emblazoned with the restaurant logo. Unlike McDonald's, Talent Camp participants get six days of activities as opposed to five. While this extra day makes the Jollibee promotion arguably a better deal since its registration is only slightly higher than what is charged for the "Kiddie Crew" (₱500–600 or $13–15) it is still pricey enough to exclude many ordinary families from enrolling.

When considered in tandem, probably what is most striking to me about these day-camp promotions is not so much the fact that kids are subject to such a direct, almost captive, form of marketing or that supervision is mostly provided by restaurant employees; rather, what stands out most vividly for me is just how conventionally accepted these offerings are in both concept and practice. At a time when McDonald's and other top chains appear on the defensive throughout much of North America and Europe about the ethics of promoting their menus and restaurants to impressionable youth, it seems quite a throwback, if admittedly somewhat quaint, to encounter manifestations of fast food outreach where such principled concerns have so little conspicuous influence.

To be sure, the popular appeal of the McDonald's "Kiddie Crew Workshop" and Jollibee's "Kids Club Talent Camp" reveals some of the underlying discontinuities that continue to characterize global fast food's variegated impact across diverse local contexts. Indeed, the wholesome image that both chains work so diligently to cultivate among Filipino families is still pretty much understood at face value by most of those promoting and participating in these respective day camps. Throughout the archipelago, fast food is still commonly viewed as a special treat that adults and kids can variously enjoy with little or no concern about its non-gustatory implications. Such notions are particularly resonant when delivered in a restaurant environment replete with elaborate playground equipment, toy giveaways, and bright and bubbly corporate mascots.

The unease or outrage that many Americans feel about industry marketing directed at children just does not readily transfer in the same way to the Philippines. Nationwide, matters of economic survival and basic well-being represent much more pressing issues for everyday households. Against this backdrop, it is hardly surprising that concerns about the ill-effects of child-centric fast food promotions lack any real sense of urgency at the local level. While it remains to be seen if such day camps will continue to elude the kind of criticism that precipitates a major retooling much less outright cancellation, I suspect they will persist in one form or another into the foreseeable future given Jollibee's and McDonald's effectiveness in sustaining lasting brand loyalty.

## FAST FOOD BIRTHDAY PARTIES

The considerable sway of corporate fast food holds over young Filipinos and their families is reflected in various ways beyond the aforementioned day camps, targeted marketing efforts, kid meal prizes, and television shows. Arguably one of the most direct and memorable expressions of this influence emerges during restaurant-sponsored birthday parties. Like other aspects of contemporary Philippine life, the roots of these childhood celebrations can be traced back to the American colonial period (1898–1946) where the commemoration of kids getting one year older became an increasingly pervasive custom for families and households nationwide. Despite some modest to significant differences in terms of etiquette and cuisine, most key elements of Filipino birthday parties would appear entirely familiar to American audiences.

Accordingly, fast food–affiliated birthday parties in the Philippines do not deviate much from what is offered by restaurant chains throughout North America. Indeed, both indigenous and multinational quick-service eateries throughout the islands have food, cake, decorations, goodie bags, and fun and games available for purchase in a variety of package deals. Perhaps predictably, both Jollibee and McDonald's have developed nearly identical party options to help local families commemorate these special events. Not to be outdone, Pizza Hut, Shakey's Pizza, KFC, and several other popular chains now offer similar all-in-one deals as a way to attract those with young children and remain competitive with the country's leading restaurant brands.

Since the 1990s, offerings of this sort have become mainstays of the Philippines' fast food scene even as they remain beyond the financial reach of most everyday households. Expenses can easily run upward of several thousand pesos depending on the party's size, theme, and duration. In this way many ordinary families are effectively priced out of this type of celebration. Despite the relatively steep costs of hosting this kind of event, however, it is not uncommon for young Filipinos of less affluent means to attend one of these get-togethers at some point or another as guests.

Based on my own ethnographic observations in San Fernando and Dagupan City since the 1990s, it seems that kids and parents overwhelmingly prefer Jollibee over its main competitors when it came to holding children's parties. Just about every Saturday or Sunday that I patronized Jollibee, some sort of birthday celebration would be under way. Either that or restaurant staff were busily preparing for or cleaning up after such festivities. Rarely did I encounter this kind of weekend revelry when visiting a McDonald's or other Jollibee rival.

To accommodate minor gatherings like these, most Jollibee, McDonald's, and other fast food chain locations in the Philippines contain separate party rooms partitioned away from their general dining areas. Besides birthday celebrations, these on-site facilities are often made available for other special occasions including confirmation and graduation parties. Renting them out is typically done on a first-come, first-served basis. When not in use, they simply serve as additional restaurant seating. Not only do these banquet areas accommodate dozens of guests, they usually feature a range of amenities to liven up festivities including karaoke systems, bubble machines, colored lighting, and mirrored disco balls.

For children's birthdays, party rooms are typically festooned with all manner of streamers, banners, and balloons. These adornments invariably reflect the gender-specific theme selected by the get-together's hosts. Most decorations feature a coordinated color scheme of sorts alongside some corresponding cartoon imagery. For example, in 2016, Jollibee offered a range of themed party packages including those based around *Hello Kitty*, *Batman*, and *Jollitown*. Quite often some type of colorful centerpiece or backdrop is crafted out of party decorations to create an area for the collection of birthday presents and distribution of goodie bags.

As a general rule, the more elaborate the celebration, the higher the associated costs. Until recently, booking these type of events for the hosts either required a lengthy phone call or in-store visit. Nowadays, party preparations are much less inconvenient as arrangements can be handled almost entirely online. Beyond signing a formal contract or paying a deposit, practically all of the food and event planning can be accomplished in a matter of minutes via company webpages. This sort of convenience and standardized party options mirrors the fast food format in more ways than one.

Fast food birthday parties hold particular appeal for parents and others willing to shell out this kind of money. Splurges of this sort not only create lasting family memories, they also help liberate the hosts from many of the small details that go along with throwing a successful birthday. Indeed, on the day of the event there is really little for parents to do beyond just showing up as most food and event preparations are already taken care of. Restaurant staff not only decorate the party room, they even take the lead in terms of coordinating simple party games and entertainment, providing the hosts ample time to tend to children and guests.

In some package deals, fast food employees will also make a surprise appearance as the company mascot. Whether portraying Jollibee or Ronald McDonald, those crew members brave enough to assume these roles must exhibit some measure of caution since this part of the celebration usually occurs toward the end of festivities when kids are more than slightly rambunctious after servings of cake, soft drinks, and assorted junk food. On more than one occasion I have witnessed youngsters forcibly remove the oversized head of a costumed character.

Clearly, as one of the few locally accessible venues capable of accommodating a sizable number of parents and children in clean and comfortable surroundings, fast food restaurants fill an important gap in municipal retailing for those looking to host kid birthday parties outside of the home. Besides perhaps select mall food courts or video arcades, no other retail spaces address this burgeoning need for middle-class families. Certainly, none offers the kinds of party package deals provided by McDonald's, Jollibee, and various other chain eateries. With the possible exception of the aforementioned day camps, no other industry offering better exemplifies the fast food experience for young Filipinos than restaurant birthday parties. Unlike these types of celebrations in the United States which have waned in popularity since their heyday in the 1980s, fast food birthday parties in the Philippines still retain a considerable amount of cachet with children and families alike.

Again, it bears reiterating that relatively few everyday Filipinos are able to experience these get-togethers firsthand as the guest of honor. The associated costs of such celebrations are effectively too much for most household budgets. Many kids and teens, however, do attend these festivities at one point or another when invited as guests by their more affluent peers. In this way, direct exposure to corporate fast food within the context of birthday parties is still somewhat limited aside from some novel attempts to engage a wider national audience with bold new approaches. The following case from one of the Philippines' top homegrown chains reveals just how such efforts can assume a rather ambitious character in terms of reach and objectives.

## BIRTHDAY BALLADS

In 2006, as linkages between quick-service eateries and birthday celebrations in the Philippines showed no signs of weakening, a multi-pronged marketing push by the aforementioned restaurant chain Goldilocks took such connections into an entirely new and inventive direction. This unexpected development entailed the commissioning of a new pop single by company executives as a viable and decidedly Filipino alternative to the enduring standby "Happy Birthday to You" (Valsino 2006). Long known for its baked desserts and point-and-order meal selections served cafeteria-style, the homegrown Goldilocks maintains hundreds of locations across the Philippines and even a few overseas branches mostly in California and Canada. Among other things, the bakeshop has few peers when it comes to creating delicious pastries and elaborate made-to-order cakes that have become standard fare at birthday celebrations nationwide.

In a move that garnered its fair share of media attention, Goldilocks management enlisted the talents of Warner Music Philippines and original Pilipino music (OPM) female artist Nina to commemorate the restaurant's 40th anniversary in 2006. What resulted from this collaboration was "*Araw Mo*" (Your Day), a heartfelt ballad performed in the sentimental style that remains popular among local music lovers of all ages. In publicizing the song Goldilocks' marketing director, Pinky T. Lee, told a national business daily, "Our research findings say that Filipinos celebrate their birthdays with Goldilocks. However, we discovered that we don't have a birthday song that we can call our own. That's why we came up with the idea of… a birthday song that we can share to all Filipinos" (Valsino 2006).

Both the accompanying music video and Goldilocks' commercial which features ordinary folk singing "*Araw Mo*" serve as almost textbook examples of the traditional OPM tropes of unabashed sincerity and earnestness. Besides working with some mobile content providers to develop an "*Araw Mo*" ringtone for cellphone users, a reasonably priced CD of the song and promotional video was sold at all Goldilocks' locations for a limited time. While "*Araw Mo*" became a moderate hit, it never quite lives up to "Happy Birthday to You" as the go-to composition that guests sing right before wishes are made and candles blown out. Still, it does represent a savvy marketing tool to showcase both the restaurant's popularity among Filipinos as well as evoke aspects of both national and brand identity across multiple media platforms.

As Lee goes on to elaborate, "Like in the song, we don't think we need to extensively place our name, Goldilocks, to bring the message across. Goldilocks is already part of the community and part of every Filipinos' lives. We all know that Goldilocks and Filipino families already have an established relationship. The song is just bringing this relationship further." So, even as "*Araw Mo*" falls short of its lofty intentions of supplanting "Happy Birthday to You"—which is still the most performed song of all time worldwide—it does showcase Goldilocks in a novel way just as it reinforces associations between birthdays and chain restaurants in the popular consciousness.

## NOTES FROM A 2006 JOLLIBEE BIRTHDAY PARTY

To add some ethnographic granularity to this section, it is probably useful to consider my own experience with fast food birthday parties in the Philippines. Such commentary not only helps sketch out some of what goes on at this sort of gathering but it also adds more resonant detail to many of the findings presented throughout this chapter. To this end, the account presented below is mainly rooted in the fieldnotes I typed up immediately following a birthday celebration in July 2006 that was held at a newly constructed Jollibee on the outskirts of Dagupan City. Indeed, with the exception of a few name changes, these fieldnotes are presented pretty much verbatim as they were recorded in my laptop. In part, this accounts for the somewhat choppy writing style.

The sleek and modern eatery was situated along a major highway near the municipality of Calasiao. Practically all of the vehicles traveling north from Manila pass by this restaurant before entering Dagupan City proper. In fact, for many years it was the most visible landmark that greeted visitors to the city besides the nearby concrete arch adorned with images of *bangus* and other municipal symbols. Like most other standalone fast food establishments in the Philippines, this Jollibee boasts a party room capable of accommodating dozens of guests. Its climate controlled ambience and modern amenities offers partygoers a welcome respite from the noisy clamor of highway traffic and ill-effects of a tropical rainy season ratcheting up in intensity.

Before delving more deeply into these kinds of observations, it is important to note that I not only participated in these festivities as a guest but also helped sponsor them. For this reason, certain background details are provided to set the scene for the descriptions below. Providing clarification in this way helps avoid any undue confusion that would render parts of what I document as unnecessarily obscure.

Given my longstanding friendship with my research assistant Mario and the family and neighbors living in and around the household where I stayed off-and-on during my local fieldwork in Dagupan City beginning in 1997 and continuing over subsequent decades, I was able to befriend quite a number of Filipinos who, with few exceptions, always treated me with considerable warmth and understanding. Their cordiality was genuinely appreciated considering I doubtless committed many inadvertent faux pas as a cultural outsider still trying to negotiate the complexities of a culture not my own. Like other anthropologists living and working abroad, I could not help but harbor feelings that my presence was sometimes only marginally tolerated by those around me.

The sense of gratitude and indebtedness that I felt toward these acquaintances who mainly resided in the *barangay* Bonuan Boquig made Mario's request to help throw a party quite easy to accept. Ostensibly to commemorate the birthday of a neighborhood preschooler but in reality more a celebration among close neighbors, I began to think of this get-together as a thank-you gesture of sorts. From what Mario said it had been quite a few years since a party like this had been thrown.

The party was for Moho, the youngest and arguably favorite child of those living in the houses surrounding his family's printing press. Even though most residents were tenants to his landlord father—who by the way was gracious enough let us pass through his property each day to get to the nearby jeepney stop—the child was still endearing enough in mischievous sort of way to garner favor. Partly as a way to repay my neighborhood friends and partly as a way to observe firsthand intersections between childhood and corporate fast food, I agreed to assume some of the cost of underwriting this festivity. In fact, Mario and I ended up handling most of the arrangements that went along with throwing the get-together at the new Calasiao Jollibee restaurant. If truth be told, I probably put in more work for this particular party than I did for my own kids' birthday celebrations back home.

In concrete terms, this meant choosing the birthday theme/decorations, bill of fare, and party time/date. We worked closely with Gian, a young man with an infectious personality, who served as our primary contact in coordinating nearly all aspects of party planning and preparation. Like most college-age Jollibee employees, he exuded the air of someone who genuinely loves interacting with customers. With his guidance, Mario and I were able to craft a selection of food and drinks from the menu and dessert options available that partygoers of all ages would hopefully find appealing.

I suppose what stands out most about our pre-party dealings with Gian and other Jollibee staffers was just how highly structured the entire process turned out to be. Only a few of the questions posed to us did not come directly from a corporate playbook that Gian seemed to carefully guard. After deciding on one aspect of the party, he would immediately reference a prepared script concealed within a sleek three-ring binder for the next question. Anything that veered outside of this narrow range of options did not seem to make it into the party agenda. While such exchanges felt somewhat artificial, they did fall within the margins of other fast food interactions I have had in the Philippines. If I had any concerns that the birthday would become some tightly regimented affair, these worries would prove mostly unfounded.

## JOLLIBEE BIRTHDAY PARTY, CALASIAO, PANGASINAN, JULY 22, 2006, 9:00–11:30 AM

The party was originally booked from 9–11 am but guests were running late. There is supposed to be an additional ₱500 fee for each extra half hour but luckily the Jollibee waived this in our case. Also, the party was contracted for only 30 guests but 41 (21 adults and 20 children) showed up. Again the Jollibee staff was very gracious and allowed us to pay for the additional guests with no problem.

Mario and I left Bonuan early to touch base with the Jollibee personnel and make sure everything was in order. Many of the guests Mario invited arrived at his house by 7:30 am. To expedite travel to the party Mario made arrangements for a jeepney to shuttle guests from Bonuan to the restaurant and back again once the party was over. The driver also showed up early, around 8:00 am.

On the way to Calasiao, I received a text message on my cell phone from Gian, the Jollibee assistant manager in charge of the party. It read:

> "gud day…ds s gian…d party area of jobee ca£asiao s nw redi…see u £8r… tnx sir TY…"
> sent: 22-July-2006
> 08:50 46

My response back was:

> "OK w are already at mayombo (a nearby Dagupan barangay). C U."
> sent: 22-July-2006
> 08:51 49

When we arrived at the Jollibee, the party room was all prepared. As we approached restaurant staff was spraying Lysol air freshener out of aerosol cans. The rented space was practically immaculate. The walls and ceiling were decorated with balloons, pennants, and pictures of the Jollibee mascots. By the party room entrance, there was a folding table set up with two sign-up sheets taped to the surface. One was for adults and the other for children. This is Jollibee's way of discreetly keeping track of the number of party attendants. Also on the table were a stack of adhesive name tags to be worn by the children.

Inside, Moho's birthday cake was already on display. It was from Pedrito's Bakeshop, a local bakery, known for their pastries and bread. The cake was in keeping with the circus theme that we had originally selected, featuring Jollibee figurines in big top attire as decorations. Paper placemats and party hats lay flat on all of the tables. Gian later informed me that it took the staff almost an hour to prepare the rented space.

As we waited for nearly half an hour for the other guests to arrive, Gian and his female assistant donned party vests embroidered with colorful balloons and the Jollibee mascot.

The party room looked out onto the restaurant's sizable parking lot. A group of six or seven street kids dressed in tank tops, shorts, and flip-flops, played *boguy*, a game very similar to hacky sack. Instead of a small leather pouch filled with pellets, *boguy* players kick around a stack of peso coins wrapped tightly in plastic and secured with a rubber band. The sack flies around almost like a badminton shuttlecock. Throughout the party, the street kids watched the goings-on inside with a keen interest. Many pressed their faces to the plate glass leaving smudges.

Throughout our wait, the party room's sound system blared out a continuous loop of songs by the Black Eyed Peas interspersed with disco versions of children's favorites like "The Wheels on the Bus" and "Happy Birthday to You."

By 9:30 am, the guests from Bonuan had arrived and the festivities got underway. There was a general feeling of excitement among the attendants as many had never attended a Jollibee birthday party or eaten at this particular restaurant. Most dressed up for the event.

Throughout the party, Gian acted as the host and emcee. He talked through a wireless microphone that seemed to be stuck on echo. Mostly he spoke in Tagalog punctuated by English. In a way, he reminded me of a talk show host ala Phil Donahue, sticking the mike in guests' faces asking if they had anything to say to Moho. Most attendants simply said, "Happy Birthday Moho."

The first order of party business was the invocation. Gian asked me to lead it but I deferred. A neighbor of Mario's eventually volunteered and delivered a short invocation, ending with the Lord's Prayer.

After this, Gian thanked me "for choosing Jollibee Calasiao Drive-thru" to hold the party. At several points throughout the morning, I was recognized for co-hosting the birthday. Each time I was referred to as "Sir Ty."

Next, Gian introduced the guest of honor, Moho. The little boy sat atop a chair during these opening remarks. Gian asked Moho if he had anything to say to the party attendants. His only reply was "thank you Mama."

With the initial comments out of the way, the party games began. Most involved some type of race pitting two teams of five against one another. Again, it was Gian who directed these activities with the help of his assistant. All of the winners received a small bag of Jollibee novelty toys. Spectators screamed enthusiastically for each game participant.

The first game was called "Bring Me Something." It was not unlike a scavenger hunt or "Let's Make a Deal" whereby players had to deliver to Gian an item he had requested. Most of the things he asked for were commonplace like a tube of lipstick or a .25 centavo coin. The first to do so would win a prize bag. Basically, the game involved the mothers frantically digging through their purses for the requested item and giving it to their children to quickly run it up to Gian. This game only lasted for 5 minutes or so.

The next game was the "Caterpillar Race." Here two teams of five children lined up in single file in front of a pair of chairs. At the count of three, the head of each line raced around a chair and returned to their line to pick up a teammate who held them by the waist. The duos then went back around the chair and retrieved another player. This pattern was continued until the entire team made it around the chair like a caterpillar. This game was over in less than ten minutes.

After the Caterpillar Race, it was the grown-ups turn to participate. The first adult game was called "S.O.S." It involves two teams of five contestants racing up to a chair one at a time, shaking their hips to spell out "S.O.S.," circling the chair, dancing again, and finally tagging the next in line. The S.O.S. game culminates with the final contestant sitting on a balloon until it pops. Of all the games, this was by far the most popular one of the morning. The kids really thought it was hilarious to see their mothers and grandmothers dance somewhat suggestively. When the balloons were popped, everyone screamed excitedly. As a crowd favorite, this game was played twice. Altogether, it lasted some 15 minutes.

Next, Gian went around with the microphone asking kids to say "Happy Birthday Moho" for as long as they could. In this game, kids would say the phrase, holding on to the last syllable of Moho's name for 10–20 seconds before running out of breath. At this point, many of the children became disinterested in the games and left the party room to play on the restaurant jungle gym also known as the "Jolly Kiddie Land." Throughout the rest of the party kids would come and go between the playground and the party room.

The final game was one for the adults called the "Plate Game." I actually volunteered to play this one. Here two teams of five had to race around a chair one by one while holding five Styrofoam plates at various points on their bodies—one between their knees, one under each armpit, one between the neck and shoulder, and the final one held like a fan. After one lap is completed, plates are passed to the next contestant to transport around the chair. Like the "S.O.S. Game," the "Plate Game" ends with a participant sitting on a balloon. Again there was lots of cheering and screaming accompanying this game.

At this point food was served. The menu package we selected included a one piece Chicken-joy (one piece of fried chicken with rice and gravy), an order of Jolly Spaghetti, a Yum! Hamburger, a small Coke, and a Hot Fudge Sundae. All menu items were brought out individually on orange Jollibee trays by the restaurant staff. It took almost 30 minutes to serve all of the dishes. Clearly, for many guests, this was way too much food to eat at one sitting. Jollibee employees soon began handing out plastic bags so that attendants could take home what they didn't eat. Best I could tell, more than half of the food served was taken home in doggie bags.

The music continued to thump throughout lunch. When Moho accidentally knocked over his Coke, a Jollibee crew member was there in less than a minute to mop it up.

As lunch was winding down, Gian asked the kids if there was anyone special they wanted to see. They all screamed "Jollibee!" He smiled and told them that Jollibee would soon appear.

In the meantime several pre-adolescent boys transformed the game area into an impromptu dance floor. As hip-hop music filtered out through the stereo, they took turns break dancing. I was really impressed by their ability to pop and lock, do handstands, and spin on their heads.

All at once, Gian interrupted their dancing to announce that Jollibee was about to appear. The dancers cleared the floor and all of the kids moved to the front of the room. Gian cued a Jollibee theme song on the sound system, saying "It is time for Jollibee to show you his talents." He then had the children count to ten and out came Jollibee from the restaurant utility room. Among all the fanfare, Jollibee made the rounds dancing, giving high fives, and posing for pictures.

In their excitement, many children couldn't resist grabbing his stinger or punching his stomach. A few of the smaller kids were obviously scared of the oversize bee; some even cried. On two occasions, Jollibee's chef's hat fell off, eliciting rounds of gleeful laughter. The highlight of Jollibee's appearance was when he performed a choreographed dance to his theme song. Roars of laughter ensued when he shook his tail in the face of a teenage girl.

When it was time for Jollibee to greet Moho as the guest of honor, the little boy was nowhere to be found. Apparently, the Jollibee was somewhat overwhelming and scary to him. It turns out he was hiding in the jungle gym during the entire Jollibee performance. An older neighbor girl eventually had to coax him out of his hiding place before he would agree to meet the giant mascot. When word got back to the party that Moho was hiding, the Jollibee leaned against a door frame, pretending to sob hysterically.

Finally, with much reassurance, Moho was placed in the arms of Jollibee. All of the guests sang "Happy Birthday" to him and then the lighted birthday candles were extinguished. Then the Jollibee pantomimed three birthday wishes to Moho. With Gian acting as translator, the Jollibee hoped Moho would;

1. Grow up to be healthy
2. Grow up to be strong
3. And finally, come back to Jollibee next year to celebrate his fourth birthday

Everyone applauded. At this point, it was announced that the party was over. Guests departed the restaurant clutching take-out bags, party favors, and balloons. Unfortunately, we ran out of time to cut the cake. So, we had to transport the boxed confection back to Bonuan.

After everyone left, Mario and I hung around to settle the bill. The Jollibee staff was very accommodating even though 11 additional guests showed up. While the paperwork was being finalized, crew members filled large garbage bags with the party refuse. The street kids outside began frantically tapping the glass and pointing to leftovers that they wanted. The Jollibee staff would not permit me to take them food but I was allowed to give them the last remaining party balloon.

With everything in order, we thanked Gian and returned to Bonuan. Later, Mario informed me that everyone had a great time. They were all trying to figure out how much it cost to pay for the party.

The get-together described above expands and reiterates much of what was presented throughout this chapter about industry efforts to reach Filipino families and children. No less significantly, it also adds various ethnographic textures to the growing influence of corporate fast food over young Filipinos through increasingly elaborate chain-sponsored birthday festivities. Several findings from this 2006 celebration warrant additional comment and consideration as they enhance understanding about how restaurant birthdays are viewed and experienced locally.

First, although much of the birthday activities followed a predetermined script that presumably came straight out of Gian's company playbook, he and other crew members were willing to deviate from this agenda when circumstances changed. For example, little was made about the unexpected overflow of guests that showed up to the party room even though this was well above the number previously agreed upon. We were not penalized for this minor breach or for the fact that the party both started and finished late but simply allowed to pay for the excess guests. While the standardization of fast food in the Philippines and elsewhere seemingly offers few opportunities for impromptu decision-making, this sort of accommodation suggests a degree of latitude on the part of restaurant staff when it comes to working outside of the strictures of fast food's "iron cage" (Ritzer 2004:28).

Second, while only touched upon tangentially, the status of quick-service eateries as gathering spots for local street kids became readily apparent at Moho's party. Not just in Calasiao but across the Philippines, Jollibee and other fast food establishments serve in this capacity for a variety of reasons; none the least of which are their centralized locations along busy corridors and the steady stream of customers with spare change or uneaten food filing in and out pretty much all day. For the most part, dealings with homeless children are accepted as an unavoidable aspect of urban life.

At least that was my impression from observing partygoers and Jollibee staffers on the morning of the birthday party. These youngsters were tolerated up to a point but not allowed to receive extra food or available leftovers from hosts or guests. Their presence on the periphery of festivities produced, at least for me, a strange dichotomy. While it is all too easy to draw some type of allegorical meaning about the socioeconomic inequalities pervading Philippine society based on the juxtaposition of our party and the street kids outside, such possibilities do little to assuage the conflicted feelings of disconnect and self-reproach I experienced about sponsoring a private celebration near so much conspicuous hardship.

Third, celebrations of this sort represent a deeper elaboration of fast food's status as a special treat or novelty for most everyday Filipinos from poor or working poor households. While emerging as increasingly common features of daily life in the provincial Philippines, these restaurants and their offerings persist mostly as the domain of those with at least some level of affluence. For local families who struggle to make ends meet, visiting Jollibee on a regular basis remains something largely unfeasible. Doubtless this is why, as I noted in Chapter Three, many of Mario's neighbors assumed it was my birthday when we had some Jollibee take-out delivered to his house by motorcycle in July 2005. Even as fast food remains cost-prohibitive for many ordinary Filipinos, rare is the pre- or grade-school student who is neither unfamiliar with Jollibee, McDonald's, and other brands nor unaware of their birthday promotions.

## FAST FOOD AS MARKERS OF GENERATIONAL IDENTITY

Just as corporate fast food maintains a conspicuous presence in the urban fabric of most towns and cities in today's Philippines, so too does it loom large over the symbolic landscapes and lived experiences of Filipino children, whether school aged or younger. Based on information presented throughout this chapter, it seems readily apparent that few kids living throughout the Visayas, Mindanao, and Luzon are able to elude the persuasive influence of popular restaurant brands. Whether through chain-affiliated advertising, television shows, summer day camps, birthday celebrations, and the like, national and international fast food companies have done much to appeal to the sensibilities of Filipino youngsters. Without overestimating the scope of the industry's marketing prowess, there appears little that concerned parents can do at this stage to effectively insulate their kids from the direct and indirect impact of quick-service eateries.

Indeed, the Golden Arches, Jollibee, and other top restaurant brands now wield considerable sway over the consumer and dining preferences of families and children across the islands. These ventures not only serve as powerful vehicles for the spread of global consumerism and Western pop culture in previously under-tapped markets, they also work to corporatize numerous aspects of the childhood experience. Unlike other parts of the world where industry efforts to reach those in and approaching grade-school have been significantly curbed or phased out altogether, such developments have yet to occur in the Philippines in a substantial way. With corporate fast food more or less viewed as an ordinary aspect of Philippine life by those with some level of affluence and considered as something of a novelty or special treat for those from poor and working poor households, the prospect of a similar reevaluation of kid-centric marketing efforts appears highly unlikely for the foreseeable future.

Such concerns have distinct bearing on matters discussed in Chapter 5. What follows is an examination of changes to the Philippines' national health profile that has unfolded in parallel with corporate fast food's continuous rise over the past 35 years. While increased consumption of this style of dining is but one of several factors contributing to some of the deleterious health effects now plaguing the country's healthcare apparatus, American-style chain restaurants do stand as some of the most visible and accessible purveyors of Western lifestyles and consumption patterns among today's Filipinos.

# Chapter 5

# Jollibesity?

## *Intersections of Fast Food, Health, Nutrition, and Obesity 2000s–2010s*

No matter how much influence corporate fast food exerts in shaping consumer sensibilities and commercial preferences in today's Philippines, it probably goes without saying that its most direct and, in some ways, insidious impact relates to the way it informs prevailing dietary habits and health outcomes. As is the case in other advanced developing countries, its aggregate effect on local individuals and households ranks it alongside the consumption of those other calorically dense and highly processed snacks, convenience fare, and sugary soft drinks promoted by industrialized food companies (Albala 2014).

A shift away from traditional eating behaviors and dining preferences to those based around established Western diets has not only accelerated notably as chains like McDonald's and Jollibee emerged as a viable force in Filipino lifeways in the 1990s but also represents a major health concern for dieticians, physicians, and others working in the Philippines healthcare system (Matejowsky 2008). In this way the country is undergoing a process of "nutrition transition" that is plaguing public and private health systems in many advanced less developed countries (Popkin 1993). Significantly, such changes have contributed to a rise in medical conditions previously only associated with Western lifestyles such as Type 2 diabetes, obesity, high blood pressure, and hypertension. Further complicating this emerging health profile are various other factors including increased sedentary lifestyles and technological dependency, insufficient exercise, and deficient or seemingly contradictory nutrition information (Popkin and Gordon-Larsen 2003).

While such changes in the Philippines' health profile would have been difficult to anticipate in previous decades given the long-standing problems of under- and malnutrition that plagued the country's healthcare apparatus, they are now some of the most pressing issues facing diverse populations across the archipelago and throughout the non-Western world (Albala 2014:172). At the macro-level, the increased weight gains and their ancillary effects can be viewed as part of the "globesity" epidemic whereby populations previously grappling with issues on one end of the medical spectrum centering around problems of undernutrition quickly find themselves at the cusp of a major new health crisis where issues of overnutrition come to the fore.

Beginning in the 1990s, when the effects of newfound economic prosperity began taking root locally, obesity rates gradually edged upward. More recently, this problematic trend has both accelerated and expanded in scope. A concomitant decline in problems of hunger and undernutrition only serves to throw prospects of a population suffering from pronounced weight gains into even more stark relief. By 2005, the proportion of Filipinos with BMI categories of overweight and obesity, classified as a BMI higher than 25 (Gibson 2005), stood at 21 percent for males and 28 percent for females (World Health Organization 2008). When obesity, defined as a BMI of over 30, is considered alone, 1 percent of males and 2.7 percent of females conform to this ranking (World Health Organization 2008). These figures seem likely to intensify as new lifestyle options become increasingly available to everyday Filipinos.

Indeed, according to the Food and Nutrition Research Institute (FNRI), an organization that conducts periodic surveys about local health practices and outcomes, three out of ten Filipino adults are now obese (Ramirez 2015). This figure represents a notable increase of 14.5 percent, since only 16.6 percent of islanders suffered obesity in 1993, compared to 31.1 percent in 2013 (Ramirez 2015).

Speaking anecdotally, I can only state that with every return visit to the Philippines since first travelling there in 1994 the number of overweight and obese individuals seems to incrementally grow. Thinking back to my initial stay in the islands some two decades ago, I seldom encountered Filipinos with high body mass indexes (BMI). Even among locals boasting some level of material affluence, it was rare to see folk carrying around extra weight. This seeming dearth of people on the heavier side was at the time somewhat dislocating for me. Coming from a country like the United States and a state like Texas where, even in the 1990s, overnutrition and its secondary effects represented a pervasive health issue thanks in part to the widespread availability of inexpensive fast food and expansive eating habits, it seemed rather strange to visit a place where the vast majority of individuals were either slender or not quite underweight.

Adding another layer of complexity to the Philippines' dealings with aggregate weight gains is the fact that so many ordinary Filipinos view carrying around some extra pounds as not necessarily problematic. In truth, many consider being heavy or modestly overweight as outward indications of individual prosperity and/or happiness. Such positive affiliations are partly rooted in those long-standing problems of under- and malnutrition that plagued parts of the country for much of the 20th century. Within contexts where getting enough food remains an ongoing challenge, it is typically only those with some level of affluence who are perceived as "fat." These skewed associations continue to linger throughout much of the provincial and urban Philippines even as nutritionists, medical professionals, and others struggle to craft a consistent message on health, diet/nutrition, and weight. I know that many of my Filipino friends and acquaintances from Dagupan were pleasantly baffled by why so many Americans seemed obsessed with dieting and bodyweight.

To date, government health agencies have been slow to recognize, much less actively respond, to the challenges of rising weight gains. At best, their efforts at addressing overnutrition and related trends have entailed raising awareness about healthy lifestyle choices via select public education initiatives. Given that these strategies have only recently been introduced, it is really too early to assess their effectiveness at positively influencing local dietary habits.

In the meantime, it is worth noting that the impact of increased weight gains are not really specific to any one segment of the population. Unlike previous decades, where obesity and overweight were primarily concerns of those with some affluence, the associated ill-effects of this growing problem are less narrowly defined. Indeed, this shift toward overnutrition has broad implications across Philippine society, since it affects nearly all socioeconomic strata, albeit to varying degrees. Perhaps most troubling is its growing impact on the health and well-being of children and young adults. Clearly, these groups are most vulnerable to the long-term health repercussions of being overweight. The fact that the country's demographic profile reflects a relatively young population, with some 35 percent of Filipinos aged 14 years or younger, makes these figures all the more disconcerting.

Recent FNRI findings provide some clarification in this regard. Between 1989 and 1998, the overweight and obesity rates for preschool children remained low; hovering somewhere below 2 percent. By 2013, these figures had steadily risen to a more troubling 4.9 percent (Ramirez 2015). For children aged five to ten, the prevalence of overweight and obesity approached 6 percent in 2003, before dropping slightly back down to 5 percent in 2013. Such positive outcomes for this demographic cohort, however, were not replicated in the next age bracket comprised of preteens and teenagers. The prevalence of obesity and overweight among those aged 11–19 years grew by 2.5 percent from 5.8 percent in 2003 to 8.3 percent in 2013 (Ramirez 2015).

While empirically based studies seeking to establish corporate fast food's role in rising obesity among Filipinos remain hard to come by, notions that fast food's increased availability has played only a minor role in this emerging trend are easy to dismiss. Significantly, the head of the Philippine Association for the Study of Overweight and Obesity, Dr. Augusto D. Litonjua, alludes to this as he blames rising obesity in the Philippines on "malling," a practice he defines as "spending the day in shopping malls and eating at fast-food restaurants" (Mydans 2003).

Although fast food consumption is only one factor driving up obesity and obesity-related conditions worldwide, it remains a dynamic agent in the popularization of Western culinary systems, especially in advanced, less developed countries like the Philippines. The adoption of new dietary practices and nutritional regimes in what was once called the Third World has contributed to increased incidences of chronic medical disorders among indigenous populations that until recently were mainly associated with developed societies. Misconceptions about fast food's nutritional value currently present serious obstacles to governments and health agencies learning to effectively combat the growing implications of populations increasingly subject to the effects of globesity. As previously noted from my own research in Dagupan City, Pangasinan, only 5 percent of 161 surveyed college students characterize fast food's dietary value as nutritionally deficient or unhealthy (Matejowsky 2009).

No less significant is the fact that Jollibee, McDonald's, and other leading chains do not place a high priority on publicizing the nutrition information of their products. Unlike recent developments in the United States and Europe, there has been no comparable push in the Philippines by consumers, policymakers, or health advocates calling for increased scrutiny of fast food's nutritional value. Far from secretively withholding data on calories, fat content, and daily recommended dietary allowances, industry players have received almost no encouragement to actively disseminate this kind of information.

Despite the problematic and wide-ranging health issues this increased intake of nutritionally deleterious fare raises, and public debate about the real and potential ill-effects of corporate fast food among everyday Filipinos remains rather muted. Such apparent indifference or lack of concern effectively parallels the reactions of local parents and families to industry marketing efforts toward children as discussed in the previous chapter. In a sense, it also reflects just how matters of food and foodways are largely absent from national debates beyond those making sure citizens get enough to eat food. The only time I remember citizens actively protesting manifestations of corporate fast food in the Philippines entailed an incident whereby municipal officials entered into a lease agreement with Jollibee to commercially develop part of a city plaza into a restaurant site (Matejowsky 2000:296).

The lack of public and/or corporate engagement on this matter may simply reflect the fact that up until recently, problems of overnutrition were generally recognized as peripheral to the nation's basic health needs. As a developing country, the Philippines faces myriad social, economic, and political issues that clearly have a more immediate impact on the everyday lives of Filipinos. With so many other concerns, the need to actively publicize nutrition information has not been injected with any real sense of urgency. Of course, just how much local eating habits would change if fast food nutrition information was more readily available is still open to question. Strictly speaking, it would be a good first step in creating a more informed consumer population given the now widespread popularity of fast food.

If fast food consumers and producers in the Philippines are increasingly confronting these types of questions, it appears that the country's fast food industry has not yet felt sufficient pressure to change operating practices in any major way. Unlike the recent experience of leading fast food operators in United States and Europe, Jollibee, McDonald's, and other popular chains in the Philippines have yet to incorporate healthy menu items into their signature bills of fare, much less adequately provide consumers with nutrition information about their signature cuisine. The salads, fruit selections, and other light fare now available at many Western quick-service eateries have yet to make a real appearance on the menu boards of national and multinational chains throughout the Philippines.

By the late 2000s, the only major fast food brand in the Philippines to embrace a more transparent policy toward the nutritional and caloric content of their particular bill of fare was McDonald's (Datinguinoo 2005:16). This operational shift mirrored recent changes adopted by the Golden Arches in the United States and Europe that emerged in response to increasingly public calls to disclose dietary information. Yet, even as McDonald's began taking steps to make such data accessible to Filipino diners, their efforts were implemented in rather covert ways. Any reluctance to publicize this content more directly is surely understandable seeing as increased consumer awareness about such issues runs the risk of adversely affecting the company's bottom line. It is entirely plausible that customers would shy away from McDonald's upon discovering that its signature Big Mac, for example, contains more than 430 calories and 16 grams of fat (Datinguinoo 2005:16).

So, before this standardized dietary information finally appeared in select publications and on the company website as it is today, it was initially only available in printed form on the back of the paper tray liners that restaurant counter staff utilize when assembling food orders. Few diners were aware of this new development as McDonald's did not widely publicize it. Arguably, fewer still would think to look for such potentially useful information on the reverse side of a disposable tray liner that was almost invariably bound for the trashcan. Indeed, alongside other table refuse, patrons would simply just discard these rectangular paper sheets that eateries use for simple advertising without ever really knowing what was printed on the back.

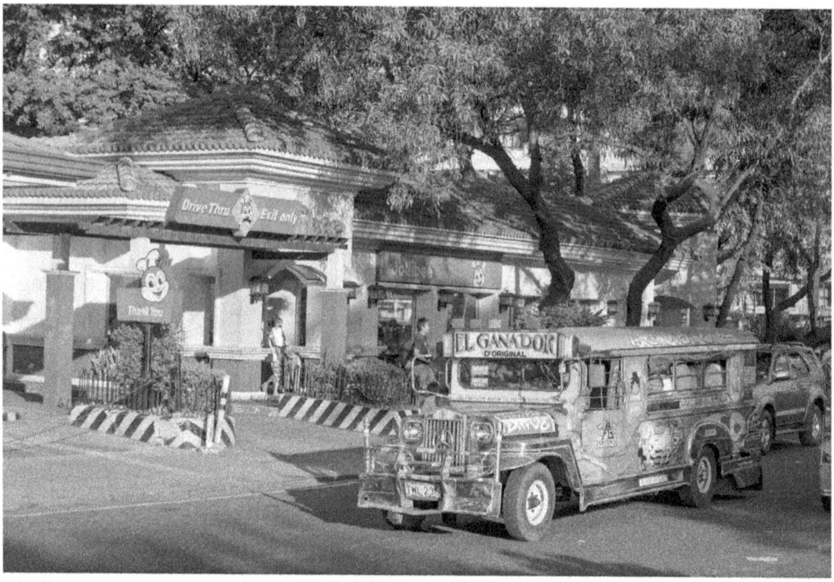


**Figure 5.1 Jeepney at Jollibee, Manila, Philippines.** © iStock.com/holgs.

Over the years Jollibee has found much success in duplicating key aspects of McDonald's restaurant operations. While replicating, the Golden Arches has paid dividends for the company in various respects, one area where Jollibee has not actively followed its main competitor's lead is McDonald's practice of publicizing, albeit in a low-key way, the calories and fat and sodium content of its popular dining selections. Even though Jollibee performed laboratory analysis of its menu items just like McDonald's (Datinguinoo 2005:16), the Philippines' top fast food chain has, thus far, avoided making its findings public. That said, select nutrition and caloric information can be found online, particularly on diet and health websites. Even if such information becomes more publically accessible, it seems that it would have little effect on the brand's long-standing popularity. Seemingly, there is now little to dissuade diners from patronizing Jollibee, McDonald's, and their various competitors.

Building off such notions, the book's final chapter will offer a synopsis of my key findings as well as some concluding thoughts on how future developments within chain restaurant operations will likely unfold over the near and long terms. However, preceding this conclusion is my final personal vignette documenting a memorable 2006 Jollibee encounter in San Fernando City.

# Conclusion

## VIGNETTE THREE: A PERSONAL ACCOUNT FROM THE FIELD, JOLLIBEE, SAN FERNANDO CITY, LA UNION, WEDNESDAY, JULY 26, 2006, EVENING

After several weeks in the Philippines shuttling back and forth between my two bases of operation in Dagupan and San Fernando City, I find myself grappling with what I can only describe as an increasingly acute case of isolation. While not exactly debilitating, this undeniable homesickness has me counting down the days until I can finally wrap up my research and begin preparations for the long journey home. For some reason, the initial sense of excitement that accompanied this second trip to the islands in two years has quickly dissipated into a kind of brooding funk, leaving me feeling lonely and out-of-sorts.

Unable to shake this melancholy, I worry that it may have inadvertently complicated my ability to collect data and negotiate the daily rigors of ethnographic research during this current stint in the field. I guess being away from my wife and young kids for almost an entire month has exacted a greater emotional toll on me than I would otherwise expect. While always a part of my fieldwork experience, this period of separation from the comforts and familiarity of home is emotionally taxing to say the least.

Exacerbating matters is the fact that the rainy season is now in full effect. The incessant downpours that started over a week ago, coupled with intense levels of humidity that leave nearly everything I own damp and musty, casts a pall over almost all aspects of local life. Here in San Fernando City, street flooding is rampant, making getting around by jeepney or foot all the more challenging. Even with an umbrella and rain slicker, I cannot venture far from my hotel without getting partially or completely drenched. One of the worse aspects of this time of year is that the air becomes so dense and heavy-laden with moisture that accomplishing even some of the simplest tasks turns problematic. For example, keeping laundry reasonably fresh assumes new levels of difficulty within this sodden air since line drying clothes is now next to impossible. With tropical humidity approaching peak levels, it takes almost a week for a pair of denim jeans to fully dry.

Under such dreary conditions, the prospect of leaving my hotel room each day becomes more and more difficult to face. I consciously stay busy during downtimes by working crossword or Sudoku puzzles and reading *Game of Thrones* novels. Compounding such gloominess is the fact that this time of year also coincides with the local cold and flu season. Almost everyone I encounter is either sick or getting over something. Those fortunate enough to elude illness are still a bit morose or moody given the prevailing circumstances. So far, I have been lucky in avoiding ill-health thanks to generous applications of hand sanitizer.

Since my hotel in downtown San Fernando offers so little in the way of room service, I am compelled to take my meals at one of several nearby eateries. Given the limited number of available choices and inconsistent hours of operation, I am probably patronizing the city's fast food restaurants a little too much. Whatever the local Jollibee, Chowking, KFC, and McDonald's lacks in healthy menu options, they more than make up for in decent surroundings and friendly service. In this regard, I am probably most partial to the second Jollibee that opened a block or so from the city's public market complex. It is usually less raucous than the chain's flagship location situated across from the town plaza.

This evening I am using the restaurant more as a casual hangout than a place to eat. I figure the Jollibee's well-lighted dining area and the friendly vibe makes for a better writing spot than the dark and dismal confines of my nearby hotel room. Plus, I am hoping that being around other people helps assuage whatever feelings of dislocation that are currently dogging me. The three-block walk to the eatery is an unforgiving exercise in remaining dry. My socks and shoes are the first casualty given the excess run-off that spills along downtown street curbs and onto the sidewalk like whitewater torrents. Roadway intersections are particularly tricky in this regard as they necessitate a requisite amount of nimbleness to avoid the sometimes ankle-deep pools of standing water. Lugging a cumbersome backpack with only a small travel umbrella for protection makes such efforts all the more challenging.

Once I reach the Jollibee, I am relieved to find no shortage of available seating. A brief inspection reveals the place to be about two-thirds occupied. It is surprising that the restaurant is not at full capacity given the bad weather outside. I assume more people would rather hunker down inside an establishment with bright and cheery fixtures than brave the unrelenting elements outside. Tables and booths are filled with an assortment of students, families, and government office workers grabbing a bite before the commute home.

After placing my order of rice and fried chicken at the restaurant counter, I amble over to an unoccupied table near the store entrance. Like their workmates behind the counter, restaurant staff exudes an air of professionalism that I come to expect from the Jollibee chain as they perform menial tasks such as busing tables and assisting diners. I unload my drenched backpack on an empty chair and deposit my wet umbrella under the table. Thick drops of rain pelt the plate glass with an intensity that obscures details of the busy street scene outside. Automobile lights and silhouettes of umbrella-touting passers-by are half-discernible amid the heavy summer shower. Until I am experiencing them directly, I tend to forget just how intense the rain can fall here along the coastal areas of Northern Luzon at this time of year.

As customers enter and leave, a growing puddle of rain begins to accumulate near the store entrance. Pretty soon, it gets it to the point where this wet patch can no longer be ignored. A restaurant employee is dispatched with a mop and bucket to sop up the excess water lest it spreads totally unimpeded. Once he sufficiently dries the area, he is joined by a uniformed security guard armed with a roll of duct-tape and several disassembled cardboard boxes. The pair works together affixing these flat rectangular sections to the floor with strips of the durable adhesive. Presumably their efforts serve as a stopgap measure to keep the entryway as clean and dry as possible. Over the course of my dinner, this makeshift flooring will extend nearly all the way from the entryway to the Jollibee service counter. It is difficult to gauge how successful this improvised layer of protection is in soaking up rainwater. By the time I depart, it is completely sodden and covered in the dirt and footprints tracked in by unsuspecting customers. In a way, it seems more susceptible to accidental falls in this dilapidated state than if staffers simply place a safety sign warning customers to use caution when coming and going.

Over the restaurant sound system a succession of heartfelt pop ballads plays. The lack of upbeat tempos or lighthearted subject matter, coupled with the constant downpour outside, does little to buoy my spirits. Among these oversentimental selections are Steve Perry's 1984 song "Foolish Heart," Stephen Bishop's hit from the *Tootsie* soundtrack "It Might be You," and a tune called "Paint My Love" by a Danish soft rock band that I suspect few Americans are even remotely familiar with called Michael Learns to Rock. No matter how many times I visit the Philippines, these three tracks never seem to wane in popularity. They are played in heavy rotation on the radio, in stores, and elsewhere alongside more contemporary Top Forty fare as if released only recently. Incidentally, I notice that the classic Steve Perry version of Journey rarely receives airplay nowadays in the Philippines since local recording artist and Journey tribute band alumni Arnel Pineda assumed lead vocal and touring duties for this definitive AOR group in 2007. Perhaps in its own small way this serves as another example of Filipinos' knack for indigenizing American influences into something new.

Unpacking the contents of my Chickenjoy from the Styrofoam container, I take a moment to savor the aromatic steam rising off the dollop of white rice and wing and thigh of heavily battered fried chicken. This combination exudes a smell that proves as comforting as it does flavorsome. Besides these main items, my combo meal also includes a small serving of brown gravy and soft drink. Over the years, I have learned by observing other Jollibee diners how to properly consume this type of fare. It basically involves tearing off individual strips of meat with my fingers and lightly dipping them in the gravy. Eating fried chicken in this way seems entirely unnatural to me. Growing up, I would eat the chicken straight off the bone, my hands and fingers getting completely greasy in the process. My inclination is to saturate the rice with brown gravy and consume this staple item by the forkful. Again, this approach appears beyond what is socially acceptable for most Filipino diners. The Chickenjoy's crispy outer skin is as golden and crunchy as the tender meat it conceals is succulent and juicy. In this way, the steamed rice offers a nice counterpoint to such savory fried fare.

After finishing my meal, I walk over to a wash station situated just outside of the on-site restrooms. The tap only produces a stream of cold water just as the soap dispenser provides dabs of anemic hand gel. I do my best to clean the greasy chicken residue from my hands and fingers. The wall-mounted hand dryer is inoperative, forcing me to fling the excess water from my hands onto the floor. Feeling somewhat self-conscious, I return to my seat and clear aside the tray and leftovers to make room for my spiral notebook. Unsurprisingly, the cover and pages are a bit soggy. The ink smears as I jot down some fieldnotes about today's largely uneventful happenings.

Writing away, I pretty much lose myself in my own stream of thoughts. After a while I begin to sense a presence just beyond my field of vision. I can feel someone approach and then hover outside my personal space, waiting for me to look up from my journaling. When I finally raise my head to acknowledge his or her presence, I see that it is a Jollibee store manager. Smiling, he politely asks if he can take my tray. Sporting a necktie and short sleeve dress shirt on which a large "I ♥ Jollibee" button is affixed, he comes across as well-meaning and if slightly anxious.

If truth be told, I am genuinely relieved that this is all he wants. For the briefest moment, I fear he came over to discover why I was furiously scribbling away in a notebook. This has happened on one or two occasions in the past, leaving me slightly paranoid about my public journaling even though I am not doing anything improper. While his offer to bus the table seems innocuous enough, I suspect that he has some ulterior motive given the way he lingers about after I pass him the tray. Such suspicions are confirmed a moment or two later when he clutches a large ledger to his chest.

"Sir, how was your meal tonight?"

"It was great. Thank you for asking"

"Sir, would you mind answering a few questions about your dining experience at Jollibee La Union branch two?"

"Ok, sure."

"Thank you, Sir. Sir, my name is Han. I am the store manager."

"Nice to meet you Han."

At this point he slides into the seat directly across from me. Any attempt on my part to remain inconspicuous is now pretty much gone. I can feel the eyes of other diners as well as those working behind the counter trained on us. As Han leafs through the ledger looking for an empty page to record my answers, I put away my pen and notebook so he has room to write. My hunch that this exchange will be entirely scripted is confirmed once he begins reading aloud from a typed sheet of questions. He rarely deviates from this paper questionnaire throughout the duration of our chat.

Right off the bat, he requests my name and address. I pause for a moment and think of how to best respond. Such personal details are something that invariably leads to confusion here in the Philippines just as they sometimes do in the States. My last name is as uncommon as it is difficult to both pronounce and spell. For many Filipinos, this invites all variety of misunderstanding. Even with my fellow countrymen, it takes some effort to adequately enunciate and clarify my name when meeting strangers for the first time. Compounding matters is the unfortunate fact that neither my surname nor Czech heritage readily conforms to local expectations of what a genuine "American" should be. Over the years I have been told in the Philippines that my first name is more "Chinese" than "American," while my last name cannot possibly be "American" since it is clearly "Russian." To expedite matters, I fish out my business cards and furnish Han with one, telling him, "All of my contact information is on here. You can just put down my university address."

He glances at the printed script on front before flipping the card over to find only blank space. Looking up he asks, "You are a doctor?"

"Yes, I teach in Florida."

From the look on his face, it seems he doesn't know what to make of this. How much of this has to with my name or occupation is unclear. Han then proceeds to ask what I think about Jollibee's menu, level service, and overall condition of the store. It is on this last point where he kind of asks some leading questions such as "Isn't it clean?" While I respond with nothing but accolades, the next part of the survey initially throws me.

"Who is your best in smile?"

"Best in smile?" I ask.

"Yes, which team member here at Jollibee La Union branch two is your best in smile?"

Best I can tell, this means who is your favorite Jollibee employee? So I answer "Han." He seems genuinely touched by this response. Building off such positive vibes, I also say nice things about him when he asks, "How do you rate your store manager's performance?" He thanks me for answering his questions, stating that the feedback will help make the store improve service. After an awkward pause, I feel compelled to say something to end this encounter both decisively and affirmatively.

"Where did you get that button? Can I have one?"

Han touches the pin-back self-consciously, replying softly, "These are for staff only."

This seems to do the trick as Han hurriedly departs. Immediately, I retrieve my notebook and begin scrawling down details from this interaction. Unlike the humdrum matters I was writing about beforehand, my conversation with Han offers enough revelatory nuggets that I feel are worth documenting. Having a Jollibee employee ask me questions about fast food operations in the Philippines rather than the other way around is an irony that is not entirely lost on me. With the tables seemingly turned, I can only chalk it up as one of those leftfield occurrences that occasionally emerge during ethnographic fieldwork. At the very least, my completion of Han's consumer survey provides some insightful details into those matters Jollibee deems important and useful when it comes to the consumer dining experience.

## FAST FOOD PHILIPPINES

During the past 35 years, corporate fast food has made considerable strides in establishing a viable presence in towns and cities throughout the Philippine hinterland. The proliferation of these eateries, alongside the foodways, nutritional regimes, and consumer sensibilities they promote, has altered the lived experiences of Filipinos in myriad ways. Information presented over previous chapters documenting the encroachment and operational aspects of quick-service restaurants in two tertiary cities in Northern Luzon—Dagupan City, Pangasinan, and San Fernando City, La Union—speaks to the variegated impact of this style of dining maintains as it continues to hold sway across varied domains of Filipino life.

Such findings are rooted in a diverse range of data elicitation techniques including semi-structured interviews, consumer surveys, and participant-observation. Collectively, they assume a particular level of granularity by dint of the autoethnographic approach I also employ throughout this account of fast food globalization. My ongoing research efforts in the provincial

Philippines, coupled with a recurring if slightly excessive patronage of these dining establishments across successive fieldwork sessions, has afforded me a useful vantage point from which to observe and document various changes in the cities' respective fast food scenes dating from the 1990s onward. With anthropological experiences in both communities extending back some two decades, this work benefits from the kind of reflexive and longitudinal perspectives that adds insights and ethnographic textures which a more straightforward critical food analysis would likely miss.

Indeed, when findings from preceding chapters are considered altogether, it is difficult to imagine a more pervasive and highly adaptable retail format operating within the commercial mainstream of today's Philippines. The influence of McDonald's, Jollibee, and other global and homegrown chains is now so far-reaching that for most everyday Filipinos it appears entirely ubiquitous and commonplace. In a nation of over 103 million with a significant segment living and working abroad as OCWs and *balikbayans*, there are few areas of local life that remain beyond the extensive reach of this ubiquitous style of dining. The iconic corporate logos, sleek signage, and child-friendly mascots are arguably as omnipresent now in the Philippines as they are in most parts of the United States and Europe. Yet, even as this American-style food phenomenon continues to hold sway at the community level, it would be erroneous to suggest that its impact over Filipino modernity is expressed with uniform intensity.

Some of the changes engendered by this continuing restaurant expansion—particularly those informing the architectural character of local cityscapes and steady rise in national overweight and obesity rates—are nothing if not entirely conspicuous. Based on these recent developments, it is difficult to overlook the subsequent impact that nearly four decades of corporate fast food growth has had on the real and material aspects of Filipino lifeways, especially in urban areas. In terms of aesthetics, since McDonald's first came on the scene in 1981, the urban fabric has assumed a much more cosmopolitan, corporatized, and in some ways sanitized character as American-style chain eateries work to redefine the street-level morphologies of built environments. Today, it is difficult to travel through either downtown Dagupan or San Fernando City without encountering some direct manifestation of corporate fast food.

Other changes appear much less tangible and discernible. To wit, the impact of this style of dining over prevailing notions of neo-patriotism, postcolonial resistance, and consumer expectations about service, taste, and lifestyle more readily approaches the abstract and ideational. While qualitative factors like these become more obvious when teased out within the context of consumer surveys and/or personal anecdotes, their onset is often so gradual that they invariably suffer in comparison to the visible immediacy of many other routine expressions of corporate fast food. Yet, no matter how observable and measurable, these alterations to the composition of Filipino modernity have now become so ingrained into the schema of everyday life that they can hardly be seen as anything all that exceptional or out of the ordinary.

For example, local food and foodways have undergone notable expansion in recent decades to gradually include popular Western staples such as hamburgers, French fries, pizza, and fried chicken. Today, such dishes actively approach, if not actually stand alongside, the more traditional fare based around rice, fish, pork, and fresh fruit selections within the Philippines' culinary canon. Without overestimating the significance of this ongoing transformation, it is clear that while Filipinos have incorporated this Western-style cuisine into their established eating habits and culinary practices, they have done so on their own terms. This kind of gastronomic assimilation reflects a long-standing penchant among Filipinos for appropriating and reimagining outside influences to produce something viable and new.

As a country located somewhere within the nexus between East and West, the Philippines has long been receptive to the trends and lifestyles emanating from abroad. The penetration of national and international chain eateries—first into Metro-Manila and other major metropolitan centers, followed by their emergence in provincial towns and cities of the Visayas, Mindanao, and Luzon—has variously altered the contours of Philippine modernity. Thanks in part to the visionary leadership of Jollibee's Tony Tan Caktiong and McDonald's George Yang and the entrepreneurial efforts of hundreds of local franchisees, numerous spheres of national life have undergone slight to significant changes with the launch of U.S.-style fast food outlets.

Similar to how the introduction of American basketball, surplus military jeeps, and other externalities from the United States has been irrevocably transformed over the years into something new and deeply emblematic of Filipino culture such as the venerable Philippine Basketball Association or passenger jeepneys, so too have aspects of corporate fast food undergone similar processes of indigenization at the local level. While Jollibee's rise to national prominence is largely predicated on replicating McDonald's global success, the Philippines' top restaurant brand has come to enjoy additional cachet as both a vibrant symbol of neo-patriotism and postcolonial resistance vis-à-vis the United States, in general, and Golden Arches, more specifically.

Such developments have advanced to the point where most of the fast food features Jollibee and other homegrown chains now share with their Western antecedents are those occurring at the structural-institutional level (Ram 2004). Whether in the United States or Philippines, virtually all of today's quick-service eateries maintain a highly standardized and regimented assembly-line production system alongside a basic uniformity in restaurant layout and signage. The tightly regulated franchise system favored by McDonald's and other popular restaurant brands whereby daily restaurant operations are handled by local contract firms significantly figures into this area of corporate fast food, as well.

These organizational details have not only proven adaptable across diverse geographic and cultural milieus, they also establish the parameters and contexts in which expressions of fast food production and consumption take place. Perhaps more than anything else, it has been these operational traits—pioneered and refined by the Golden Arches and its various rivals over the years—that bolster arguments suggesting an inextricable link between corporate chain eateries and processes of unilateral global homogenization. When considered in this light, such features appear widely consistent across various fast food scenes just as they are familiar to global diners whose appreciation for this popular eating format belies significant differences in nationality and cultural heritage.

Yet, as evidenced by findings from the Philippines, in general, and Dagupan and San Fernando City, more specifically, this operational uniformity in corporate fast food only goes so far. Transcending the material components of quick-service eateries is an aspect of chain restaurant operations that more readily accommodates local tastes and trends. Unlike the underlying sameness encountered at the structural-institutional level, it is at the expressive-symbolic level where various types of heterogeneities and discontinuities in fast food production and consumption emerge (Ram 2004). Within this less rigidly defined context, manifestations of globalization and localization interface and influence each other in multiple ways. The linkages between these domains have grown increasingly interpenetrative, developing a clear capacity for the production of new and sometimes quite singular results. In this way, indigenous chain restaurant owner-operators and their clientele are able to engage corporate fast food with varying degrees of agency and indigenization.

As in other global markets, chain restaurant operations in today's Philippines are characterized by a number of distinguishing traits and idiosyncrasies that set them apart from what occurs elsewhere. Such attributes do much in defining the overall personality of the country's fast food scene just as they reflect long-standing preferences and practices within traditional Filipino foodways. Based on the enduring rivalry between Jollibee and McDonald's documented in chapter 2, it is those eateries which are most locally attuned and responsive to customer predilections that achieve success.

Accordingly, these distinctive characteristics encompass matters related to both fast food production and consumption. In concrete terms, these features prove useful in distinguishing how Filipino consumers conceptualize chain restaurants, utilize their products, and adapt to the contexts they create. Similarly, they help promote understanding about the ways in which fast food outlets emerge, operate, and engage local markets. Ethnographic details presented over previous chapters particularly those found in chapters 3 and 4 as well as the various personal vignettes—consider these various aspects of corporate fast food and elucidate both the profound and subtle ways that this popular dining fare and format is experienced in the Philippines.

In terms of consumer preference, Filipinos' established partiality for sweet flavors and ingredients rather than the tangy, if somewhat sour, tastes often emphasized by U.S. quick-service eateries is one of the reasons Jollibee has outperformed its main competitor McDonald's for so many years. Even as the Golden Arches has developed products such as the Burger McDo and Chicken McDo that resemble those of its primary Philippine competitor and, thereby, better align with the traditional Filipino palate, these items have failed to capture the appetites and imaginations of Filipinos in the same way as Jollibee fare.

Accordingly, the menu boards of global and homegrown chains across the islands have increasingly featured Filipino dishes that would likely only meet limited success if sold anywhere else. The Golden Arches' ever popular McSpaghetti, Jollibee's *Palabok* Fiesta, and Chowking's *halo-halo* are but some prime examples that come to mind in this regard. Similarly, the special emphasis attributed by many quick-service eateries to the traditional afternoon snack of *merienda* is something that is not regularly encountered in other global fast food markets. Whether in terms of college and high school students adopting dining areas as makeshift afternoon hangouts or the various desserts and light fare offered for sale during this venerated snack time, it is notable how fast food patrons and producers have integrated *merienda* into chain restaurant operations.

In terms of production, even as some restaurant brands encounter more success than others in this regard, it is clear that nearly all of the chains examined herein consciously utilize the fast food format in ways to effectively engage Filipino tastes and sensibilities. Besides creating an ambience befitting local sentiments through a soundtrack of much-loved Tagalog and Western pop ballads to the availability of party rooms featuring karaoke systems and other entertaining amenities, much thought goes into appealing to basic Filipino tastes and preferences. Again, the development of specialized menu items that jibe well with local palates as well as advertising campaigns and marketing efforts that address enduring cultural values such as an ingrained deference to families and children speak to such endeavors.

Although trying to attract families and children is not something that readily distinguishes corporate fast food in the Philippines from its American and European counterparts, it is evident that Jollibee and McDonald's strive to reach this important segment of the Filipino dining public in a manner that deeply resonates with local sensibilities even as it departs somewhat from earlier Western approaches. From the popularity of the bee mascot featured in advertisements and the television show *Jollitown* to outreach and promotional efforts such as McDonald's "Kiddie Crew" and Jollibee's "Kids Club Talent Camp," various attempts at winning the patronage of parents and kids have been implemented. In many ways, these efforts resemble those practices previously utilized by restaurant brands in Europe and North America in the 1980s and 1990s that were phased out due to parental and consumer concerns about health and nutrition alongside the ongoing corporatization of childhood.

## FUTURE TRAJECTORIES

In writing a book about the processes of fast food globalization that have transformed local lifeways in the provincial Philippines over the past four decades, it is useful to consider what factors may inform future developments within the country's fast food scene in the years and decades to come. Obviously, such efforts run the risk of devolving into uncritical speculation since teasing out prospective shifts in restaurant operations and the foodways they encompass is something laden with all types of unknowns. Bearing such thoughts in mind, I still feel confident in identifying several factors worth considering when anticipating future trajectories of how and where such developments may occur. Such ample assuredness is based partly on my years ethnographically documenting corporate fast food expansion in Dagupan and San Fernando City and partly on my familiarity with ongoing refinements and innovations within this sector of the global restaurant industry. With regard to the latter, the critical insights I have gained on this topic from teaching my undergraduate UCF class, "Anthropology of Fast Food," since 2011 have proven indispensable.

Before turning attention to such factors and their potential implications, however, it bears reiterating just how deeply enmeshed American-style chain eateries have become in the daily life of towns and cities throughout the Philippine hinterland. The amenities and products they provide have become so well integrated into established consumer expectations and lifestyles that initial concerns about the long-term success of this retail sector have long been laid to rest. For what was once considered an open question, it now seems hard to imagine how the viability of corporate fast food in the Philippines was ever seriously in doubt.

The preliminary success of McDonald's, later surpassed by Jollibee, has created a flourishing fast food scene comprised of multiple national and international eateries. Today, these operations and their loyal customer clientele represent nothing if not a significant achievement for a consumer market economy long characterized by middling, sporadic, and sometimes uneven growth. For Jollibee, the company's preeminence among Filipino diners shows no sign of slacking even as the firm expands internationally into various parts of Asia, North America, and elsewhere. The eatery's continued dominance of its main rival McDonald's remains a considerable source of national pride.

Against this backdrop, there are three areas that I feel warrant particular consideration for understanding future developments within the Philippines' prevailing fast food scene. While their respective influences may not always generate sweeping changes at the local level, they each retain a certain gravity that increasingly places them and corporate fast food within each other's specific orbits. Areas worth watching when it comes to anticipating how the overall tone and character of chain restaurant operations will be experienced by Filipino diners over coming years are: (1) technology; (2) health; and (3) increased prosperity.

## TECHNOLOGY

Although always a part of chain restaurant operations, the significant integration of digital technology into how fast food brands conduct business is clearly one sphere that will experience ongoing development in the near and distant future. Expanded availability of on-site Wi-Fi like what is offered by the country's Starbucks' operations, coupled with an increased dependency on smartphone apps including those designed for easy payment or ordering takeout or delivery, appears all but certain. In fact, Jollibee has already tested the waters in this regard having launched various gaming and advertising apps, many of which are aimed directly at tech-savvy children and teenagers. The near ubiquity of cellphones, smartphones, and other mobile devices within the theater of the ordinary, even among Filipinos of more modest means, suggests that the transformative influence of digital technology will add new textures and dimensions to the production and consumption of corporate fast food in the Philippines.

## HEALTH

While concerns over corporate fast food's ill-effects on public health have not yet reached the point where radical industry changes appear imminent, they do cast a shadow over this restaurant sector that will arguably only intensify over the years to come. Unlike recent developments in the United States and Europe, where fast food operators have taken steps—sometimes self-imposed, sometimes compelled through outside regulation—to create a more informed dining public by publicizing nutrition information and offering healthy menu options, similar efforts have failed to gain momentum locally. Even as the country's health profile continues to undergo profound reconfiguration thanks in part to encroaching Western nutritional regimes and eating habits rooted in convenience, industry leaders in the Philippines have, thus far, remained relatively insulated from any pressure to significantly alter or revise their operations.

The mounting health crisis posed by those Western-style-medical conditions falling under the umbrella term of "globesity," however, may prove too substantial to ignore indefinitely. How much this looming predicament serves as a catalyst for substantive change remains unclear. I suspect that if such modifications are implemented they will almost certainly unfold in a gradual if not somewhat superficial way. Complicating such efforts is the fact that the salads and fruit selections proffered as healthy fare in the United States and Europe are not the sort of cuisine to which most Filipinos naturally gravitate. At the very least, those efforts by American and European parents and health advocates that have successfully compelled McDonald's and its competitors to modify their operations serve as viable cases for analogous changes in the Philippines.

## PROSPERITY

Like any commercial sector, the success of the Philippines' fast food market is largely contingent upon the financial prosperity of its consumer base. As the country continues to reap benefits from a steadily improving economy over the past several years—thanks in part to significant infrastructure upgrades, labor flexibility, and decreasing redundancy and electricity prices—the financial forecast for everyday households has turned increasingly upbeat. Even as economic opportunities still elude many rural residents, these market improvements, alongside the continued stream of OCW and *balikbayan* remittances pouring into the islands, bodes well for the Philippines' fast food scene. With more and more locals possessing the kind of disposable income that makes their patronage of Jollibee, McDonald's, and other chains entirely viable, newfound pressures emerge among these rival brands to vie for this expanding clientele. This sort of competition creates a dynamism that leads to innovation and expansion.

When considered altogether, it seems that pressures emanating from the spheres mentioned above—technology, health, and economic prosperity—will exert an increasingly pronounced influence over the Philippines fast food landscape throughout both the near and distant futures. As such developments seemingly loom on the horizon, it remains evident from my analysis of corporate fast food in the provincial Philippines just how much this style of dining now transcends its global roots. For some 35 years, Filipinos have actively engaged this popular retail format, transforming both its production and consumption into something deeply reflective of local culture and foodways.

# Bibliography


AC Nielsen 2004. Consumers in Asia-Pacific. Our Fast Food/Take Away 2nd Half, 2004. Retrieved September 18, 2008: http://www2.acnielsen.com/reports/index_confidence.shtm

Active Research Center 1994. *Factbook Philippines* (Vol. 1994). Manila, Philippines.

Albala, Ken, ed. 2014. *From Famine to Fast Food. Nutrition, Diet, and Concepts of Health around the World.* Westport, Connecticut: Greenwood Press.

Appadurai, Arjun 1996. *Modernity at Large. Cultural Dimensions of Globalization* (Public Worlds, Vol. 1). Minneapolis: University of Minnesota Press.

Barber, Benjamin R. 1992. Jihad vs McWorld. *The Atlantic Monthly.* March 269(3):53–65.

Barber, Benjamin R. 1996. *Jihad vs McWorld. Terrorism's Challenge to Democracy.* New York: Ballantine Books.

Bartholomew, Rafe 2010. *Pacific Rims. Beermen Ballin' in Flip-Flops and the Philippines' Unlikely Love Affair with Basketball.* New York: New American Library.

Basa, Restituto C. 1997. *The Story of Dagupan.* Dagupan City, Philippines.

Beriss, David and David Sutton, eds. 2007. *The Restaurants Book. Ethnographies of Where We Eat.* New York: Berg.

Blim, Michael 2000. Capitalisms in Late Modernity. *Annual Review of Anthropology* 29:25–38.

Bosco, Joseph 1999. An Anthropological View of the Hong Kong McDonald's Snoopy Craze. *Hong King Anthropologist* 12:23–30.

Business Asia 2000. Cashed-up Filipinos Feast on Fast Food. Business Asia, February 11.

Carrozal, F. P. 1886. *Memoria de Pangasinan 1885. Archives of the Dominican Order, Tomo 121.* Quezon City, Philippines: Convent of Saint Dominic.

Coe, Sophie D. and Michael D. Coe 1996. *The True History of Chocolate.* New York: Thames and Hudson.

Conde, Carlos H. 2005. Jollibee Stings McDonald's in Philippines. International Herald Tribune. May 31.

Cordero-Fernando, Gilda, ed. 1976. *The Culinary Culture of the Philippines*. Quezon City, Philippines: Bancom Audiovision Corporation.

Cordero-Fernando, Gilda 1992. *Philippine Food and Life*. Quezon City, Philippines: Anvil Publishing.

Cuevas, Likha C. 2007. Jollibee's 2006 Earnings Jump on Strong Sales. Manila Times International. February 15.

Dannhaeuser, Norbert 2004. *Chinese Traders in a Philippine Town. From Daily Competition to Urban Transformation*. Quezon City, Philippines: Ateneo de Manila University Press.

Datinguinoo, Vinia 2005. *The Big Picture. iRepot. Feast and Famine. Food and the Filipino*. Quezon City, Philippines: Philippine Center for Investigative Journalism.

De Leon, Sunshine Lichauco 2013. Billionaire Tony Tan Caktiong takes Jollibee Foods Global. Forbes, January 30.

Downie, Andrew 2000. Barrio Burgers. McXperiment: Serving Billions in the Slums? Christian Science Monitor, January 26.

Economist 2002. A Busy Bee in the Hamburger Hive. If McDonald's is the Goliath of Fast Food, Tony Tan's Jollibee is its Filipino David. Economist, February 28.

Economist 2016. Acquired Tastes. A Tenacious Filipino Burger Chain Tries a Different Way to Conquer the World. Economist, January 9.

Elias, Megan 2014. The Palate of Power. Americans, Food and the Philippines after the Spanish-American War. *Material Culture* 46(1):44–57.

Ellis, Carolyn and Arthur Bochner 2000. Autoethnography, Personal Narrative, Reflexivity. Researcher as Subject. In *The Sage Handbook of Qualitative Research* (2nd edition). Norman K. Denzin and Yvonna Lincoln, eds. Thousand Oaks, California: Sage.

Fantasia, Rick 1995. Fast Food in France. *Theory and Society* 24:201–243.

Flores, Wilson Lee 2011. George Yang's Success Tip. Be Honest, Persevere and Work Really Hard. Philippine Star, December 4:N3.

Franger, Bert 1994. The Meyhane or McDonald's? Changes in Eating Habits and the Evolution of Fast Food in Istanbul. In *Culinary Cultures of the Middle East*. Sami Zubadia and Richard Tapper, eds. New York: I.B. Tauris.

Friedman, Thomas L. 1999. *The Lexus and the Olive Tree: Understanding Globalization*. New York: Farrrar, Strauss, Giroux.

Garland, Alex 1998. *The Tesseract*. New York: Viking Books.

Gartzke, Erik 2007. The Capitalist Peace. *American Journal of Political Science* 51:166–191.

Gibson, Rosalind 2005. *Principles of Nutritional Assessment*. Oxford: Oxford University Press.

Goldstein, Myrna Chandler and Mark A. Goldstein 2002. *Controversies in Food and Nutrition*. Westport, Connecticut: Greenwood Press.

History of San Fernando 1983. Souvenir Program 130th Anniversary. San Fernando, City, Philippines.

Imbong, Peter 2015. The Untold Story of how Jollibee came to Bee. Entrepreneur Philippines, January 22.

Inglis, David and Debra Gimlin 2013. Food Globalizations. Ironies and Ambivalences of Food, Cuisine and Globality. In *The Globalization of Food*. David Inglis and Debra Gimlin, eds. New York: Berg.

Jackson, Christine 1979. Ethnography of an Urban Burger King Franchise. *Journal of American Culture* 2(3):534–539.

Jing, Jun, ed. 2000. *Feeding China's Little Emperors. Food, Children, and Social Change*. Palo Alto: Stanford University Press.

Jollibee 2007. Frequently Asked Questions. Retrieved August 3, 2007 from Jollibee Web Site: http://www.jollibee.com.ph/corporate/lib_faq.htm

Kincheloe, Joe 2002. *The Sign of the Burger. McDonald's and the Culture of Power. Labor in Crisis*. Philadelphia: Temple University.

Koeppel, Dan 2008. *Banana. The Fate of the Fruit that Changed the World*. New York: Plume.

Kottack, Conrad P. 1978. Rituals at McDonald's. *Journal of American Culture* 1(2):370–386.

Kurlansky, Mark 2003. *Salt. A World History*. New York: Penguin.

Laurel, R. Kwan 2010. *Philippine Cultural Disasters. Essays on an Age of Hyper Consumption*. Pasig City, Philippines: Willing Ox Publishing.

Lee, James and Leonie Karkoviata 2001. Fast Track to Growth. Homegrown Enterprises Leverage on Proven Franchising Systems. *Asian Business* 37(12):29–36.

Lim, Benito 1997. The Dagupan Chinese. *Chinese Studies Journal* 7:16–36.

Luxner, Larry 2002. Made to Order: From Humble Beginnings in Brazil, Fast-Food Chain Bob's is Giving Global Giants such as McDonald's a Run for their Money in Latin America's Largest Consumer Market – Strategies. Latin CEO: Executive Strategies for the Americas. January.

Maréchal, Garance 2010. Autoethnography. In *Encyclopedia of Case Study Research*. Albert J. Mills, Gabrielle Durepos, and Eldon Wiebe, eds. 2:43–45.

Matejowsky, Ty 2000. The Privatization of Public Plazas in the Philippines. Three Cases from Pangasinan. *Philippine Quarterly of Culture and Society* 28(3):263–300.

Matejowsky, Ty 2006. Global Tastes, Local Contexts: An Ethnographic Account of Fast Food. In *San Fernando City, the Philippines. In Fast Food/Slow Food: The Economic Anthropology of the Global Food System*. Society for Economic Anthropology Monograph Series 24, Richard Wilk, ed. Pp. 145–159. Walnut Creek, California: Altamira Press.

Matejowsky, Ty 2007. SPAM and Fast Food "Glocalization" in the Philippines. *Food Culture and Society* 10(1):23–41.

Matejowsky, Ty 2008. Jolly Dogs and McSpaghetti: Anthropological Reflections on Global/Local Fast Food Competition in the Philippines. *Journal of Asia-Pacific Business* 9(4):313–328.

Matejowsky, Ty 2009. Fast Food and Nutritional Perceptions in the Age of "Globesity:" Perspectives from the Provincial Philippines. *Food and Foodways* 17(1):29–49.

Matejowsky, Ty 2013. The Incredible, Edible Balut. Ethnographic Perspectives on the Philippines' Favorite Liminal Food. *Food, Culture and Society* 16(3):387–404.

Meimban, Adriel Obar 1997. *La Union. The Making of a Province. 1850–1921.* Manila, Philippines: Rex Printing.

Mintz, Sidney W. 1985. *Sweetness and Power. The Place of Sugar in Modern History.* New York: Viking.

Mydans, Seth 2003. Clustering in Cities, Asians are Becoming Obese. New York Times. March 13.

Noguchi, Paul H. 1994. Savor Slowly. Ekiben. The Fast Food of High-Speed Japan. *Ethnology* 33(4):317–330.

Norton, Michael 2000. Today's Special: Happiness. New Fast-Food Joint in Haiti a Beacon Amid Gloom. Houston Chronicle, September 5.

Ohnuki-Tierney, Emiko 1997. McDonald's in Japan. Changing Manners and Etiquette. In *Golden Arches East: McDonald's in East Asia.* James L. Watson, ed. Stanford: Stanford University Press.

Paradeza, Joel 1997. Got ₱7 Million? Put up a Jollibee Store. Philippine Daily Inquirer, October 13.

Pertierra, Raul 1995. *Philippine Localities and Global Perspectives. Essays on Society and Culture.* Manila, Philippines: Ateneo De Manila Press.

Philippine Daily Inquirer 1998. McDonald's to Pursue Expansion. March 21.

Philippine Star 2008. Behind-the-Scenes of Every "Langhap-Sarap" Serving. June 26.

Phillips, Lynne 2006. Food and Globalization. *Annual Review of Anthropology* 35:37–57.

Popkin, Barry 1993. Nutritional Patterns and Transitions. *Population and Development Review* 19(1):138–157.

Popkin, Barry 2008. *The World is Fat. The Fads, Trends, Policies, and Products that are Fattening the Human Race.* New York: Avery.

Quimpo-Espino, Margie 2004. This Jolly Man Deserves his "Langhap Sarap" Success. Philippine Daily Inquirer, June 26.

Rai, Saritha 2005. India's Boom Spreads to Smaller Cities. New York Times, January 4:C3.

Ram, Uri 2004. Glocommodification. How the Global Consumes the Local. McDonald's in Israel. *Current Sociology* 52(1):11–31.

Ramirez, Robertzon 2015. Number of Obese, Overweight Pinoys Increasing. Philippine Star, July 2.

Ritzer, George 1998. *The McDonaldization Thesis.* London: Sage.

Ritzer, George 2001. *Explorations in the Sociology of Consumption. Fast Food, Credit Cards and Casinos.* London: Sage.

Ritzer, George 2004. *The McDonaldization of Society.* Revised New Century Edition Thousand Oaks, California: Pine Forge Press.

Schlosser, Eric 2001. *Fast Food Nation: The Dark Side of the All-American Meal.* Boston: Houghton Mifflin Co.

Schneier, Bruce 2003. *Beyond Fear. Thinking Sensibly about Security in an Uncertain World.* New York: Copernicus Books.

Sering, Tara F. T. 2011. The Journey of George Yang. Philippine Star, December 4:N1–2.

Sobal, Jeffery and Wm. Alex McIntosh 2008. Globalization and Obesity. In *The Globalization of Food.* David Inglis and Debra Gimlin (eds). New York: Berg.

Spurlock, Morgan 2004. Super Size Me. Samuel Goldwyn Films.

Stein, Joe 2007. The Hungry American. Foreign Fast Food Chains are Moving into the U.S. and Showing How the World Really Sees Us. Time Magazine, April 9.

Stephenson, Peter H. 1989. Going to McDonald's in Leiden. *Ethos* 17(2):226–247.

Stolicna, Rastislava 2000. Fast Food: the Global Phenomenon of Today's Eating Habits and Lifestyle. *Slovensky Narodopis* 48:305–313.

Trager, Lillian 1988. *The City Connection. Migration and Family Interdependence in the Philippines.* Ann Arbor, Michigan: University of Michigan Press.

Traphagan, John and Keith Brown 2002. Fast Food and Intergenerational Commensality in Japan. New Patterns and Old Patterns. *Ethnology* 41(2):129.

Valisno, Jeffrey 2006. Goldilocks Whips up Treat for Celebrating Birthdays Pinoy Style. Business World, July 21–22.

Van Esterik, Penny 2008. *Food Culture in Southeast Asia. Food Culture Around the World.* Westport, Connecticut: Greenwood Press.

Vistro, Jesus Victor and Crispin Reyes 2005. *Nandaragupan. The Story of a Coastal City Dagupan Bangus.* Dagupan City, Philippines: Dagupan City Heritage Commission.

Volpe, Tina 2005. *The Fast Food Craze. Wreaking Havoc on Our Bodies and Our Animals.* Kagel Canyon, California: Canyon Publishing.

Watson, James, ed. 1997. *Golden Arches East: McDonald's in East Asia.* Stanford: Stanford University Press.

Wilk, Richard 2006. *Home Cooking in the Global Village. From Buccaneers to Ecotourists. Anthropology and Material Culture.* New York: Bloomsbury Academic.

Wong, David 2007. Battling Against a Brand. Change Agent. Synovate.

World Health Organization 2008. BMI/Overweight/Obesity Prevalance. Country Comparable Data. http://www.who.int/ncd_surveillance/infobase/web/InFoBaseCommon/

Wu, David Y. H. 1997. McDonald's in Taipei: Hamburgers, Betel Nuts and National Identity. In *Golden Arches East: McDonald's in East Asia.* James L. Watson, ed. Stanford: Stanford University Press.

Zhongqiang, Jin 1999/2000. Kentucky Fried Chicken, McDonald's and Chinese Drama. *Chinese Sociology and Anthropology* 32(2):35–37.

# Index

# About the Author

**Ty Matejowsky** is an Associate Professor in the Department of Anthropology at the University of Central Florida in Orlando. In 2014, he was awarded the Association for the Study of Food and Society's Belasco Prize for Scholarly Excellence for his publication "The Incredible, Edible *Balut*: Ethnographic Perspectives on the Philippines' Favorite Liminal Food."

CPSIA information can be obtained
at www.ICGtesting.com
Printed in the USA
BVHW01*1453071217
501867BV00004B/8/P

9 780739 139882